Patient Navigation

Elizabeth A. Calhoun · Angelina Esparza
Editors

Patient Navigation

Overcoming Barriers to Care

Springer

Editors
Elizabeth A. Calhoun, Med, PhD
Health Policy and Administration
University of Illinois at Chicago
Chicago, IL
USA

Angelina Esparza, BA, BSN, MPH
ACS Patient Navigation Program
American Cancer Society
Atlanta, GA
USA

ISBN 978-1-4939-6977-7 ISBN 978-1-4939-6979-1 (eBook)
DOI 10.1007/978-1-4939-6979-1

Library of Congress Control Number: 2017933549

Printed on acid-free paper

This Springer imprint is published by Springer Nature
The registered company is Springer Science+Business Media LLC
The registered company address is: 233 Spring Street, New York, NY 10013, U.S.A.

Foreword

Since President Richard Nixon's declared war on cancer in 1971, various interventions and new technology have helped combat cancer in the U.S. and around the globe. However, the benefits of these medical interventions are not shared by all and disparities continue to exist. Health disparities driven by poverty, culture, and social injustice has kept the healthcare system out of reach for certain geographic, ethnic, and racial subgroups of the population, resulting in poorer health outcomes for them and thus greater health disparities.

Patient navigation is increasingly gaining popularity as an effective intervention to minimize disparities in cancer screening and cancer care. Navigators have successfully been used to overcome logistical barriers to care by lowering time-to-initial treatment and diagnostic resolution in cancer patients. Patient navigation programs have been widely implemented in a variety of settings, for a variety of populations, and by a variety of people with different professional and cultural backgrounds, and to improve outcomes for a variety of diseases, such as cancer, cardiovascular disease, human immunodeficiency virus (HIV)/acquired immunodeficiency virus (AIDS), asthma, and diabetes. Navigators can work with patients from underrepresented populations to address financial and insurance issues, coordinate appointments among multiple care providers, address language barriers, and train patients to advocate for themselves.

Patient navigation is both a community-based and health system-based service delivery intervention designed to promote access to timely diagnosis and treatment of cancer. The first patient navigation program was created in 1990. The program was initially conceived to increase cancer survival rates by reducing the time between a suspicious finding and resolution of the finding through diagnosis and treatment. Today, the scope of patient navigation programs range across the healthcare continuum to include screening, detection, diagnosis, treatment, and follow-up care. Patient navigation has also extended to other medical conditions beyond cancer and gained further traction with the passage of the Affordable Care Act.

The literature documents the success and results of patient navigation programs; however, few have delved into practical implementation strategies for a successful program. This book is the culmination of years of research and practical experience by scientific leaders in the field.

The authors intend the book to be used as a practical guide to creating, implementing, and evaluating successful patient navigation programs. The goal of the book is to help readers walk step-by-step through patient navigation from identifying the need for patient navigation (perhaps through community assessment) to understanding various patient navigation models, creating and implementing a successful program, training patient navigators, evaluating patient navigation programs for continuous quality improvement, and arguing for systematic policy changes that integrate patient navigators into the healthcare system. The chapters in the book elaborate on the principles of many successful patient navigation programs that have been developed and vetted for over 20 years in diverse population groups:

- Navigation is a patient-centric healthcare service delivery model
- Core function of navigation is the elimination of barriers to time care access across all segments of the healthcare continuum
- Patient navigation should be defined with a clear scope of practice that distinguishes the role and responsibilities of the navigator from that of all other providers
- Delivery of navigation services should be cost-effective and commensurate with the training and skills necessary to navigate an individual through a particular phase of the care continuum
- The determination of who should navigate should be primarily decided by the level of skills required at a given phase of navigation
- There is a need in a given system of care to define the point at which navigation begins and the point at which navigation ends
- There is a need to navigate patients across disconnected systems of care, such as primary care sites and tertiary care sites
- Navigation systems require coordination

In addition to serving as a guide for patient navigation programs, the book also discusses practical approaches to various ancillary functions which serve as a foundation for the successful implementation of patient navigation. For instance, the chapter on community needs assessments provides practical insights and discusses various toolkits to conduct an effective needs assessment. Various theories and models, including the Logic Model, are discussed to reflect how they can be used in the context of evaluating patient navigation programs. Other practical aspects such as structural readiness and psychological readiness of an organization are also discussed as effective change management strategies when an organization is in the process of implementing patient navigation programs.

While this book primarily serves as a template for patient navigation in cancer care, it can be extended to various other medical conditions including chronic illnesses. Patient navigation programs are a proven strategy to minimize healthcare disparities and it is our hope that this book will help educate and promote widespread implementation.

Harold P. Freeman
Harold P. Freeman Patient Navigation Institute
New York, NY, USA

Contents

Contributors

Tracy A. Battaglia, MD, MPH Department of Medicine, Boston Medical Center, Boston, MA, USA

Elizabeth A. Calhoun, Med, PhD Center for Population Science and Discovery, University of Arizona Health Sciences, Tucson, AZ, USA

Sarah E. Caron, MPH Section of General Internal Medicine, Women's Health Unit, Department of Medicine, Boston Medical Center, Boston University School of Medicine, Boston, MA, USA

Angelina Esparza, BA, BSN, MPH Houston Health Department, Houston, TX, USA

Linda Fleisher, PhD, MPH Department of Population Science, Fox Chase Cancer Center, Oreland, PA, USA

Yvonne Kellar-Guenther, PhD Community and Behavioral Health, Colorado School of Public Health, Aurora, CO, USA

Chrissy Liu, JD Point B, Seattle, WA, USA

Rebecca Mason, BS Center for Population Science and Discovery, University of Arizona, Tucson, AZ, USA

Molly McCoy, MPH, BS Section of General Internal Medicine, Women's Health Unit, Boston Medical Center, Boston University, Boston, MA, USA

Sumayah Nuhaily, MPH Department of Psychology, San Diego State University, San Diego, CA, USA

Elizabeth Ojo, BA University of Michigan, Ann Arbor, MI, USA

Steven R. Patierno, PhD Department of Medicine, Duke Cancer Institute, Durham, NC, USA

Betsy C. Risendal, PhD Department of Community and Behavioral Health, Colorado School of Public Health, Aurora, CO, USA

Anne M. Roubal, PhD, MS Population Health Sciences, University of Wisconsin, Madison, WI, USA

Yolanda Suarez-Balcazar, PhD Department of Occupational Therapy, College of Applied Health Sciences, University of Illinois at Chicago, Chicago, IL, USA

Patricia A. Valverde, PhD, MPH Community and Behavioral Health, Colorado School of Public Health, Aurora, USA

Kristen J. Wells, PhD, MPH Department of Psychology, San Diego State University, San Diego, CA, USA

Elizabeth M. Whitley, PhD, RN Colorado Department of Public Health and Environment, Denve, CO, USA

Chapter 1
Community Needs Assessment: Bringing Real Voices to the Health Care System

Yolanda Suarez-Balcazar

Community needs assessment is grounded in the belief that people are often the best judges of things that matter most to them, that no one can walk in someone else's shoes, and that for health care interventions to make an impact, they need to include the perspectives of the consumers [1]. Community needs assessments go beyond focusing on identifying the needs and problems of communities to identifying their assets, strengths, and capacities.

Community needs assessment has been used to improve outcomes for a variety of common health conditions including cancer [2], cardiovascular disease [3], community health [4], and mental health [5]. This chapter is designed to provide an overview of community needs assessment strategies that health care providers can use with a variety of patients in clinical and community settings in order to better meet the needs of the patients, increase compliance and adoption of health innovations, and improve health outcomes. Community practitioners and researchers alike believe that individuals are the best judges of their own health issues and are more likely to adopt and comply with recommended health interventions and become a true partner in their treatment if their voices are included on what matters most to them. *To make a significant difference in the lives of individuals and communities, their voices count on what matters most.*

Essentially, a community assessment seeks to identify a group's strengths and needs to guide in establishing priorities that impact its health status. This chapter is written for health care providers seeking to engage in a needs assessment (NA) process.

Y. Suarez-Balcazar (✉)
Department of Occupational Therapy, College of Applied Health Sciences, University of Illinois at Chicago, 1919 West Taylor Street, Room 354, Chicago, IL 60612, USA
e-mail: ysuarez@uic.edu

E.A. Calhoun and A. Esparza (eds.), *Patient Navigation*,
DOI 10.1007/978-1-4939-6979-1_1

Why should you do a Needs Assessment?

- To learn more about the needs and assets of a group or community. Community needs assessments provide a way for you to diagnose the needs of the community, supplementing your own sharp-eyed observations and experiences. They can give you detailed information from a larger and more representative group of people than you could get from observations and clinical experiences alone [1, 6].
- To get a more honest and objective description of needs from the perspective of those most affected.
- To become aware of possible needs that you never saw as particularly important or that you never even knew existed.
- To make sure any actions you take and/or program and health initiatives you develop are in line with needs that are expressed by the community.
- To obtain community support for the health actions/initiatives you will undertake. People are more likely to support and use a service/program they have identified as a need.
- To get people actually involved in the subsequent action itself.

Defining the Community or Group of Interest

Communities can be defined by:

- A common health condition of a group of individuals—e.g., breast cancer survivors who are within 1–3 years of remission.
- A shared geographical space—e.g., a group of individuals within a neighborhood or who live within a specific location.
- Demographic characteristics such as race and/or ethnicity—e.g., Latino immigrants with a specific health condition.

What is a Need?

A need denotes a gap from the perspective of the individual who is experiencing a concern or issue [1]. This is a gap between what one has and what is not available. A *need* might be specific to a particular individual, group, or community experiencing a common problem or issue that is not always universal, while a *universal need* speaks to health, food, shelter, and other basic necessities.

In essence, a need can denote:

- lack of services, benefits, necessities, or goods that are essential, from the patients' perspective, to sustain health;
- lack of affordability of the aforementioned resources;
- lack of access; and/or
- lack of satisfaction with what is available.

What is a Needs Assessment?

Witkin and Altschuld [1] defined *needs assessment* (NA) as a "systematic set of procedures undertaken for the purpose of setting priorities and making decisions about program or organizational improvements and allocation of resources. The priorities are based on identified needs" (p. 10).

In other words, an NA is conducted not only to determine the needs of a group of people, but to gather information from the patients themselves, about their values, ideas, and perceptions, in order to make decisions that benefit them. It is a useful approach to increase the impact of health interventions, uncover specific areas of need, increase the likelihood of use of health care interventions, and plan for addressing areas of need, thus increasing the likelihood of improving health outcomes in a community and among individual patients.

Figure 1.1 details a useful framework to review NA strategies for Patient Navigator programs. The phases of the model include planning for the needs assessment, identifying the appropriate strategies, implementing the needs assessment, data analysis and data interpretation, acting on needs assessment feedback, and reporting.

ACA Community Benefit Requirement

As a requirement of the Affordable Care Act, not-for-profit hospitals must complete a Community Health Needs Assessment at least once every three years to maintain their tax exempt status. This can be performed in partnership with other clinics, public health, and population health focused groups who serve the same community. Because of this federal requirement, resources and tools to complete the NA continue to be made available in order to assist organizations in creating an impactful NA [7].

Planning the Needs Assessment Before you begin the NA, you need to identify a team of individuals at your clinical setting, health care system, or local or state government that can assist and provide ongoing support and feedback. A NA is not just about selecting a strategy and method to collect data from program participants; NA requires planning, ongoing brainstorming on how the data might be used in

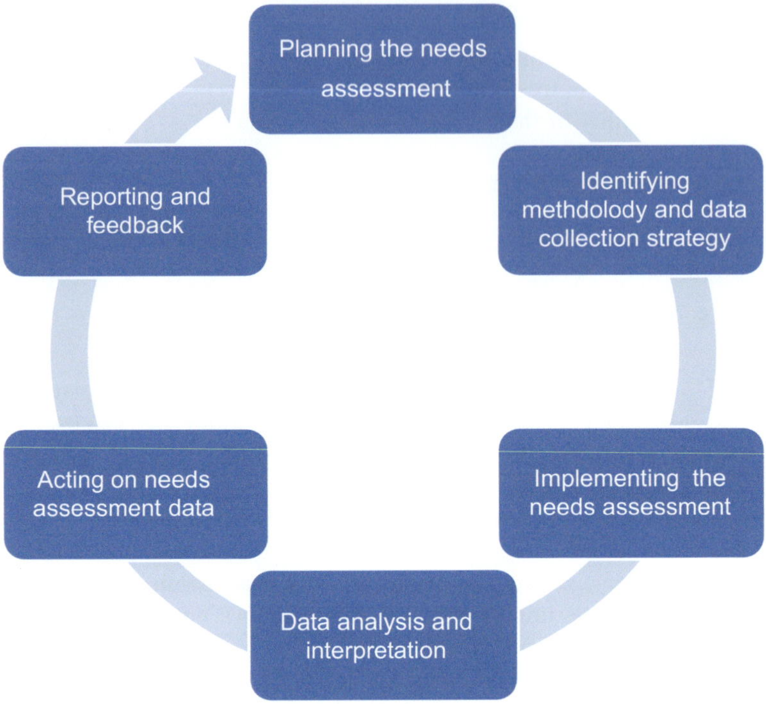

Fig. 1.1 Community needs assessment process. Adapted from Witkin and Altschuld [1] and Suarez-Balcazar, Orellana-Damacela, Portillo, Sharma, and Lanum [6]

action planning, and decision making. Witkin and Altschuld [1] and the Community Tool Box [6], suggest considering the following during the planning phase:

- What is the purpose of the NA? Why are you doing it?
- Does a NA already exist for your community? When was it conducted? Who led the effort? (The ACA requires NAs be conducted every three years, have an implementation strategy, take input from persons who represent the needs of the community, and be widely available to the public.)
- Is there a nonprofit hospital in your community that is already conducting a community needs assessment as required by the ACA? Can you partner in that existing NA effort? Who will be conducting the NA? Do they have the capacity to do so? (skills, knowledge, experience, time, resources?)
- What are the information needs of different stakeholders? (e.g., health care professionals, patients and their families, decision-makers, community in general). How is the data going to be utilized?

- Who will use the data? Would the team be ready to act upon the needs assessment findings? Who is interested in the NA results? A needs assessment should not be undertaken if there is no intention to follow up on the findings or act on them.
- Who is your *group/community of interest?*
  - What do you know about the community/group of interest? (Search local archives, inquire with other health professionals, and/or ask community leaders). What are their characteristics? Who are you trying to reach? Who are important stakeholders that need to be included and in what capacity?
  - What is the social, economic, health, and political history of the community/group of interest?
  - What is the relationship of the group/community of interest with the clinical setting sponsoring the NA?
  - Who are the gatekeepers and how can you obtain their support for the NA process?
  - What role will the community gatekeepers have in the needs assessment?
  - What role will the community of interest have in the needs assessment?
- What is the timing of the needs assessment? Consider the deadline for when the data/information is needed.
- What are the resources and likely scope of the NA? Consider the resources, supports, and community partners (e.g., nonprofit hospitals, local health departments) needed and available to conduct a NA. These resources will vary depending on the type of NA and scope of the project. Some expenses that you need to consider include: incentives for participants; refreshments/food for meetings or focus groups; staff overtime; cost of printing materials, protocols, surveys; cost of data entry and data analysis, transportation to and from meetings for participants and other logistics; and translation of materials, among other costs.
- How well do you know the program/service or clinical setting sponsoring the program or providing the services? What is their credibility in the community?

Before moving into the next phase, you need clear answers to the above questions while paying particular attention to the *purpose* and *potential participants*. Develop a needs assessment plan (e.g., responsible people, timeframe, resources available, and potential uses of the data) as you move forward. For an example of a need assessment, please see: UIC Mile Square Health Center Community Needs Assessment.

Identifying the methodology and data collection strategy There are several strategies for conducting a NA, many of which can easily take full chapters by themselves. Among the most common strategies reviewed in this chapter include: (a) surveys/questionnaires, (b) interviews, (c) focus groups, and (d) public forums/town hall meetings. The following is a brief description of these needs assessment strategies. Surveys typically involve quantitative data analysis methods.

Interviews might involve both qualitative and quantitative analyses, while focus groups and public forums/town hall meetings involve, for the most part, qualitative methods.

Surveys/Questionnaires

What is a Survey?

The purpose of a survey is to collect information that represents the views, personal opinions, or attitudes of individuals [1, 6]. Surveys are especially useful when gathering data from a number of people in a short period of time. Surveys come in many different forms, such as structured and standardized surveys/questions, surveys created as part of a particular needs assessment, and surveys with a combination of specific rating scales and open-ended questions. Surveys can be administered in small groups or one-on-one. Survey data can also be collected online, via telephone, or mail. Surveys usually require short answers from respondents (Yes/No, Likert-type ratings scales that reflect degree of agreement, satisfaction, difficulty, need, or degree of importance).

Recommendations for Designing a Survey/Questionnaire

- Depending on the purpose of the survey, create your own survey questions or search for a standardized survey protocol that measures what you want to measure. In either case, keep the survey's *purpose* in mind when formulating or selecting questions.
  - Clearly specify what information you need and how you might ask about it.
  - Clearly identify the components/parts of the survey, and its main content/areas (e.g., demographic information, satisfaction questions about outpatient services for people with cardiovascular diseases, level of agreement regarding health care professionals' quality of treatment).
  - Search for surveys that have already been developed that measure what you want to measure. Try contacting local public health departments, other nonprofit hospitals, and/or public health researchers to see what measures worked well for them.
- Decide whom you will survey (i.e., your target population) and choose an appropriate sampling method.
  - Clearly specify who the potential respondents are that can provide you with the needed information. Respondents are selected because they are the intended targets of the program/service to be created or modified, based on the results of the NA.

  - Who is your community?
  - How would they be reached?
  - Is the survey format the most appropriate and sensitive for the population of interest and the type of information you want to collect?
  - Ensure your sampling method will keep the sample representative of the target population. Consult a biostatistician or program evaluator who can assist with these methodology issues.

- Decide how you would like to distribute your survey (e.g., a small group survey administration, a face-to-face interview, online, or a mail questionnaire).
- Decide how and who will analyze and compile the results of your survey.
- When using existing instruments, check for cultural fit, literacy issues, and standardization with the population of interest.
- Where can you find the appropriate survey/instrument to assess what you want to assess? (Try consulting with your community health department or a University to see what is already available).
- Do you need to develop a protocol for distributing and administering the survey?
- Do you need to adapt a survey used previously?
- Is the survey instrument you selected assessing what you need to assess?

Recommendations for Developing Survey/Questionnaire Questions

- Place easier questions first.
- Check survey items for clarity and simplicity.
- Use a logical order.
- Consider the health literacy of participants, language usage, and language preferences.
- Have a colleague or team member check each item for accuracy, wording, and completeness of survey items in terms of areas covered to meet its purpose.
- Consider length of the survey. Lengthy surveys tend to produce fatigue, a pattern of responses, and/or missing data (stay within 2–3 pages if you can).
- Add/delete or modify survey items as you go through several rounds of revisions.
- Have health providers interested in the data, community leaders, and other partners review the survey.
- Make sure every survey item addresses only one question.
- Avoid double-negative items.
- Address sensitive issues or uncomfortable topics discreetly and sensitively.
- Pilot test your survey with an individual likely to share some characteristics with the actual respondents.

- Develop a well-written cover letter to accompany the survey stating the purpose of the study and what will be done with the results.
- Develop a procedure for following up with those who have not responded to the survey.

Considerations and Drawbacks of Using Surveys for the Purpose of Needs Assessment

Surveys tend to elicit socially desirable responses, especially if they are administered in small groups or one-on-one. Consider if this is likely to be the case with your NA survey. To minimize this, pay careful attention to how the items are worded, who is asking the questions, if applicable, and assure respondents that all information is confidential.

When designing a survey, consider the level of literacy and education of potential respondents. Ethnic minority populations from low-income backgrounds, individuals with low levels of education, individuals with limited English proficiency, and the elderly tend to show low response rates to surveys. These groups often have trouble with scales and structured surveys.

Recommendations for Mode of Survey Delivery

There are three main strategies for delivering the survey:

- <u>One-on-one delivery</u>: Most appropriate when low-literacy levels are likely, there is a need to read the survey to participants, the contact with the community is sporadic, and/or the community is hard to reach. Take into account the need for interpreters and translation services if respondents are likely to be non-English speakers. Note that this type of delivery of a survey requires allocation of resources including staff time and appropriate space to administer the survey.
- <u>Online survey:</u> Most appropriate for college and young adult populations. Consider the digital divide—access to computers might be limited for some populations including low-income, elderly, migrant populations and refugees, and individuals with disabilities [8]. Resources needed are minimal except for the expenses related to staff time developing the survey. Use a survey platform that allows for easy flow, allows the respondent to save changes, and is accessible to individuals with disabilities. Test your online survey before launching it. Provide the survey as a link and not as an attachment. Some commonly used survey platforms include Survey Monkey and Qualtrics.
- <u>Mail survey:</u> Tends to produce a low response rate compared with delivering the survey individually and/or in small group sessions. The low rate of response can be augmented using incentives to participants. It is a less expensive method compared to individual or small group survey administration.

Scenario 1
A local health clinic in collaboration with a hospital wants to develop a program to address the healthcare needs of individuals at risk for HIV. A 3-page survey was developed containing sensitive questions about dating, sex practices and health care. The survey is sent in the mail to single men and women in their database living in a specific geographical community of the urban city. The survey is confidential, does not ask for name or any identifiable information, and includes a $5 dollar bill and a stamped return envelope.

Interviews

What are Interviews?

Interviews are defined as conversations with a purpose [6]. They can be particularly useful when you need to know about individuals' assumptions and perceptions of activities in a given community, or to collect in-depth information on a particular topic from individuals experiencing an issue or problem. Interviews can be formally structured, semi-structured, or not structured at all depending on the purpose and needs of the project. Formally structured interviews involve an interview schedule with a list of specific questions. In semi-structured interviews, the interviewer uses an interview schedule; however, s/he can change the order of the questions and probe for further information. In unstructured interviews, an interviewer does not follow any particular schedule, but rather, uses an interview guide. Interviews can be conducted in-person, over the phone, or online (e.g., using skype, chatroom). Although the method must be chosen to fit the needs of the survey and the type of population you are surveying, sensitive information is much more likely to be gathered over phone or online interviews, but these generally have lower response rates. These methods can be more uniform than in-person interviews. However, in person interviews can generally provide more in-depth information.

Recommendations for Designing an Interview

- Identify the purpose of the interview.
  - What are the information needs and why is the interview the most appropriate strategy?
- Consider access to potential participants, time set aside, confidentiality and privacy issues, and sensitive nature of the information sought.
- Decide who should be interviewed depending on the purpose of your project.

- Decide on the interview structure and prepare the interview materials accordingly.
- Do not schedule an interview too early in the morning or too late at night.
- Consider translation and interpretation issues when planning an interview with individuals who do not have English as a first language.

Recommendations During the Interview

- Introduce yourself and your project.
- Have an icebreaker before the interview begins.
- If tape recording the conversation, ask for authorization to do so.
- Stay focused on the questions that need to be asked; however, keep flexibility in mind and probe for elaboration or pose other questions if needed:
  - Take detailed notes.
  - Show genuine interest in interviewees' responses.
  - Finish the conversation cordially and thank the interviewee.

Requesting personal narratives during the interviews: Personal narratives are individual accounts/stories of events and experiences of impact to the individual. In these narratives, an individual may recount how she experienced a disease, the impact it had on her daily life and that of significant others, and/or how she addressed the disease. When analyzing narratives, look for common themes, emerging needs, and ideas on how individuals address needs.

Scenario 2
A local hospital team conducted phone interviews with relatives of older patients who had suffered a severe stroke 3 weeks after being released. The focus of the interview was to assess the need for support, care management, management of stress, and fatigue of caregivers of stroke patients.

Resources needed for an interview mostly include health care professional's time, private space to run the interview, possibly incentives to participants, and payment of logistics (transportation for participants and translators if needed).

Focus Groups

What are Focus Groups?

The purpose of the focus groups is to provide in-depth understanding about the needs, attitudes, opinions, experiences, or expectations of a population. Focus groups seek to engage in a deep discussion about a specific topic and allow participants to share their experiences around the issue being discussed. They seek insight on a single topic. Support services such as transportation, child care, and sign language interpreters should be provided, if requested. It is recommended that you invite about 15 people in order to secure 8–10.

Recommendations for Running a Focus Group

- Explain the purpose of the focus group.
- Take questions.
- Ask participants to express their concerns and experiences about the topic of discussion.
- Have someone take notes on what participants say.
- Allow everyone in the group the opportunity to talk.
- At the end of the focus group discussion, provide a brief summary of the main issues discussed.
- Distribute any printed materials related to the topic of discussion.
- If applicable, ask participants if they would like to be part of the planning committees for acting on the results of the NA. Take participants' names and telephone numbers.
- If applicable, tell participants about the planned public forum. Circulate a flyer with date, time, purpose, and place of the planned public forum.

Resources needed for running focus groups include a meeting place, copies of any materials that might be distributed at the focus group, a note taker, and refreshments. When planning a focus group with community residents who have had very little contact with the clinic conducting the NA, it is recommended to run the focus group in a community site such as the local library, a park and recreation facility, a church or faith building, or a local community agency. Community residents may find the hospital location intimidating.

Recommended Questions for Focus Group Discussion

The following are examples of questions to ask during an informal focus group with new young mothers of children with disabilities:

- What are some supports that you have experienced when seeking health services for your child?
- What are some barriers that you have experienced when seeking health services for your child?

During the group discussion, prompt participants to talk about their personal experiences as they relate to the above issues. Make sure everyone has an opportunity to express his/her opinion.

Remember to:

- Take notes.
- Tape record meetings if necessary, and obtain approval for recording with participants and the Institutional Review Board (IRB).
- Plan for a two-hour meeting.
- Make sure everyone in the group is given an opportunity to talk (try your best to not let one person dominate the focus group).
- Provide a summary to focus group participants of what was said at the meeting at the end.

Scenario 3
Situation in which the service is not available: lack of bilingual personnel delivering programs in residents' preferred language

Latino immigrants experiencing a condition such as chronic diabetes are not utilizing a health service provided by a local hospital. A focus group conducted in the community, to which 8 Latino individuals with diabetes were invited, revealed that the service was not being used, in part, because there were not any bilingual healthcare providers at that particular hospital delivering the program. The hospital used this data to hire new staff and deliver the program in Spanish.

The Nominal Group Technique

The *Nominal Group Technique (NGT)* is a widely used technique in NA often confused with a focus group. This is a group process in which 6–8 people meet for one hour, produce a long list of ideas about an issue, and set priorities and ideas for addressing needs [1]. In contrast, the focus group seeks to engage in a deeper discussion about a specific topic and allows participants to share their experiences around the issue being discussed. While the purpose of the NGT is to formulate as many ideas as possible and prioritize them (scope), the focus group seeks depth on a specific topic.

Potential questions for a NGT process with a group of 6 women who completed a 6-month cancer treatment include:

1. Identify all aspects of your health care—preparatory, intervention, post-intervention, and follow up that you found to be satisfactory.

2. Identify all aspects of your health care—preparatory, intervention, post-intervention, and follow up that you would like to see improve.

Note that the purpose of this NGT is to identify all aspects of care that matter to women who have gone through cancer treatment.

A focus group with the same group of women, designed with the purpose of learning about the specific experiences of women as they go through treatment might ask the following questions:

1. Describe your personal experience interacting with healthcare personnel during the different phases of your treatment—preparatory, intervention, post-intervention, and follow up.
2. Share examples of support systems that have helped you deal with your treatment.
3. Share examples of barriers and challenges you experienced.

Town Hall Meetings

What are Town Hall/Public Forum Meetings?

Town hall meetings, also referred to as public forums or community forums, are large, open gatherings of individuals who are concerned about an issue or health condition and who are interested in expressing their ideas and suggestions for improving the issue or condition. Town hall meetings, depending on recruitment efforts, can easily include over 50 people. The purpose of the public forum is to gather the opinions of individuals from diverse backgrounds and experiences who share a common interest in the topic. A town hall meeting often includes a brief introduction of the issue, an overview of the purpose of the meeting, an update of what has been done to date, specific questions about the issue to discuss, and occasionally small breakout group discussions depending on the size of the group.

Recommendations for Planning a Town Hall Meeting

- Have a clear purpose of why you are having a town hall meeting and what you want to accomplish.
- Find a meeting room that is fully accessible, like a local public library or the sponsoring agency. Avoid meeting at the local hospital, if you can, as this kind of setting is often intimidating for participants.
- Reserve a large room for at least 3 hours.
- Arrange for food, interpreter services, child care, and transportation if needed.

- Post announcements on agencies' (local library, coffee shops, departments of public health, and other businesses) bulletin boards.
- Contact the local radio station to announce the town hall meeting.

To run a town hall meeting you might need a flip chart, markers, refreshments, nametags, and, depending on the size of the room and the number of expected participants, a microphone. Note that if people with hearing disabilities are attending, you may need a sign interpreter and an accessible location. If individuals who speak a second language attend, you may need interpreter services. On the posted announcements, include a phone number so that people requiring assistance can request services in advance.

Recommended Questions to Ask in a Town Hall Meeting

- What are the issues related to (the area/problem) that you are most concerned about?
- Why is this a concern/need?
- How are you affected by the issue?
- When are you affected the most?
- What impact does the issue have on your family and significant others?
- What are the consequences of keeping the issue as it is?

If utilizing breakout sessions to get more information, ask group members to discuss the following:

- What are the priorities in regards to this issue?
- What needs to be done and what can we do to address the top priorities?
  - What are the specific action steps?
  - Who needs to do it?
  - By when?
  - What resources are needed?

The smaller breakout groups will report to the larger group. The results from each breakout group can then be combined in order to move the town hall forward.

Recommendations for Running Public Forums

- If smaller breakout groups are going to be utilized, you will need a large room that will allow for round tables and/or smaller adjacent rooms. Avoid doing the town hall meeting in an auditorium.
- Identify an experienced facilitator.

- Make sure to add a few icebreakers to help people feel comfortable with individuals they do not know.
- Make sure that those who want to talk have the opportunity to do so.
- Have a note taker during the large group discussion and in the smaller breakout groups.
- Have breakout groups report to the larger group a synthesis of their ideas.
- Include a wrap up at the end of the session; discuss next steps and how the data collected will be utilized.
- Put together a report and distribute it to those who attended the session.
- Follow up on actions and feedback received.

Other Strategies

Photovoice is another strategy often used with vulnerable populations such as individuals with disabilities, teenagers, and children. Individuals are provided with cameras and asked to take pictures of things they do or see in the community that they would like to change. In one example, 7th graders were asked to take pictures at home of things they do and/or eat that make them healthy and things they do or eat that do not make them healthy. Once the pictures were printed, the children were asked to share their thoughts about the pictures, and what they could do to change habits. Their thoughts and ideas were utilized by the science teacher and researchers to help the children identify needs and set individual goals to promote healthy lifestyles [9].

Implementing the Needs Assessment

Where do we go from here? Now that common strategies used in NA have been reviewed, you need to decide which strategy will work best to accomplish your goals and which NA methods are most appropriate and suitable to your potential participants, purpose, goals, and programs. Consider the following questions:

- Who are the target participants in the NA process? Will you include all participants or a sample of participants?
- What is your sampling method?
- How and when are you collecting data? Is the protocol ready?
- What resources are available to conduct the NA?

By the time you get to this phase, you and your team will likely have a plan on how the NA is going to be implemented. The **products** of this phase include a set of tools or NA instruments and a summary of the data/information collected. This template (Table 1.1) is suggested to help you plan the implementation of the needs assessment:

Table 1.1 Implementation of the needs assessment

Purpose of the Needs Assessment: ______________________________

Target audience	How would participants be identified?	Strategy for data collection	Participant/sample selection	Resources needed	Timeframe/ When would data be collected?	Who will collect data? Where?

Data Analysis and Interpretation Analyzing and synthesizing data depends on the type of data collected—qualitative (perceptions, views, opinions), quantitative (numbers, categories), or mixed methods (qualitative and quantitative used to complement each other). If you are using structured surveys or questionnaires that require participants to use a rating scale, consider using an Excel spreadsheet or statistical software (e.g., SPSS) to summarize the results and produce descriptive statistics. Depending on the number of respondents, the types of questions asked, and types of analysis you want to produce, consider hiring a statistical consultant. However, keep in mind that most descriptive statistics of a small sample size can be done in-house.

Data resulting from interviews, narrative stories, focus groups, and public forum/town hall meetings will provide you with qualitative data. Consider looking for common themes, identification of needs, specific individual perceptions about how they are affected by a problem or unmet need, how they address the needs in their daily lives, and what alternatives and solutions exist for them. Specifically, data should allow you to answer some, if not all, of the following questions:

- What are the issues? What are the unmet needs?
- What do people think about the issues?
- How are they affected by the issues?
- Who is affected by the issue?
- When and where are they most affected?
- What can be done to address the issues?
- Why should something be done to address the issues?

Some mechanisms for analyzing qualitative data are content analysis, narrative analysis, discourse analysis, framework analysis, and grounded theory. More information on each of these methodologies can be found elsewhere [10]. We suggest consulting others (i.e., statisticians) prior to analyzing your data to avoid bias. Finally, consider using a software for analyzing qualitative data. One example of such software may include ATLAS-ti.

Taking Action on Needs Assessment

Acting on NA is an essential part of the process. Why do an NA if there is no intention of acting upon the identified needs? Data gathered from the NA can be utilized internally or externally (Table 1.2) [11].

It is important to maintain an activity log of how NA data is being used, by whom, when, and to what degree. This information needs to be shared with the community who participated in the NA.

Reporting and Feedback

Consider the following questions as you prepare a report on your needs assessment and provide feedback to the stakeholder groups sponsoring the project and those who participated in the community needs assessment:

- How should the findings be organized in a final report?
- Who should have a copy of the final report?
- What would be the best way to disseminate the final report and seek feedback and action ideas from stakeholders?
- What do you need to do to ensure and facilitate implementation of results and recommendations?
  - Who needs to be involved in planning for utilization?
  - What actions need to be taken to improve program/initiative, practices, services, and/or policies?
  - What tracking systems will allow a recording of actions to improve the program/initiative?

Table 1.2 Internal and External Uses of NA Data

Examples of internal uses of NA data	Examples of external uses of NA data
Self-reflection among health personnel Set goals to improve services, include reflections in strategic planning	Data is shared with funders, policymakers, researchers and other stakeholders
Health personnel make adjustments to programs and services	Include data in grant funding activity. Secure funding
New services and programs are created	Share data with the community and the media to call attention to health issues
Changes in practices—how existing services are delivered	Demonstrate accountability to stakeholders
Changes in policy (e.g., walk-ins policy is adopted)	Data is presented to and discussed with legislature to support the passage of a bill

- Do you need multiple versions of the report? Perhaps an executive summary and 1 page report are appropriate for specific audiences while others will want a more detailed report.
  - Make the report visually appealing. Add pictures and graphs to convey the information succinctly.
  - Make sure to include the relevant data for the audience. For some this might be a lengthy table, others may just require summary numbers.

The **products** of this phase include the needs assessment final report and a list of actions based on the recommendations resulting from the needs assessment. This information should be distributed among the individuals who will find it useful and can act upon it. Be sure to provide copies to local health departments and other coalitions who may be working in the areas identified in the report.

Context and Cultural Considerations in NA

All NA activities need attention to context and culture. Communities are infused with cultural elements that inform the way individuals define and conceptualize issues and needs, the way they live their lives, and relate to social and health systems around them. As our society becomes increasingly diverse racially, ethnically, and linguistically, context and culture have become critically important. These cultural factors may include, but are not limited to, differences in worldviews and behavioral practices, traditions celebrated, ways of learning and doing, belief systems and values that may affect how individuals define needs, and what methods and strategies work best for them. Attending to culture and context means considering the following:

- Health literacy and literacy issues in general. Consider the benefits and limitations of using visual displays. What is the most appropriate NA strategy for the population of interest given their educational level and sociocultural factors?
- Language and translation issues—appropriateness and sensitiveness of translations. Remember that it is not enough to do a contextual word-by-word translation.
- Culturally appropriate ways to reach out to participants for the needs assessment. Ethnically diverse populations may respond better to door-to-door canvassing, phone and personal interviews and surveys than mail surveys or internet-based strategies.
- When conducting interviews, surveys, focus groups, and any other NA technique that requires direct contact with participants, you must understand cultural differences in the notions of space, time, direct contact, and style of communication.
- Consider cultural differences on how individuals experience and view "health," "disability," "wellness," "recovery," and "illness."

- Consider cultural differences in the communication style and how these differences might inform behavioral patterns.
- Consider access to the devices and supports needed to participate in the NA (phone, computer, transportation to and from).
- Consider participants' understanding of the IRB approval process. The issues of confidentiality and compensation have to be carefully explained when conducting an NA. Submit your request for Institutional Review Board (IRB) approval. Take time to explain what it means when conducting NA with populations with little or no experience with IRB.
- Consider issues of accessibility of the NA (strategies, methods and protocols) when working with individuals with disabilities.
- Consider cultural fit when using standardized surveys and protocols with populations different from those for which the survey was developed.
- Consider cultural attitudes and behaviors about the purpose of the NA. People from diverse ethnic and cultural backgrounds, when controlling for education and socioeconomic status, might feel differently about participating in a survey study vs. participating in a chat room or focus group. Attitudes and beliefs about sharing private information with people they do not know and beliefs about health and well-being might influence their participation.

A Community-Based Participatory Needs Assessment Example

A community needs assessment method, which has been used successfully to identify and address the needs of various vulnerable populations, is called the *Concerns Report Method* (CRM) [6, 12–14]. This is a systematic and participatory set of strategies designed to identify health concerns, brainstorm solutions, and take action from the perspective of individuals experiencing a health condition or concern. The CRM uses focus groups, a concerns survey, and a public forum to achieve its aim. It is grounded in the principles of participation and the inclusion of community members in the earliest stages of identifying and defining concerns/needs, setting priorities, and designing intervention strategies. It has been conceptualized as an agenda setting, capacity building, and empowering approach to community needs assessment [14].

The following example describes the application of the CRM to identify the health service needs and ideas for action from the perspective of Latino immigrants.

In Sum, the Concerns Report Method:

- Involves community members in the decision-making process early on, which increases their likelihood of getting actively involved and staying involved in addressing health issues.
- Asks community members to define what they see as most important. This is information that you will not get from professionals who have not experienced the issue (concern or problem).
- Is reliable, systematic, and easy way to tap into information about the community of interest.
- Provides a useful source of information and direction for initiatives, funders, and participants.
- Helps set the agenda for acting upon the concerns/needs.
- Builds consensus and identifies not only concerns/needs, but strengths as well.

Case Study Background

A large medical group in the suburb of a Midwestern city experiencing a high rate of new Latino immigrants undertook an initiative to improve the health services provided to the community [12]. The initiative began with a partnership between a local hospital, a community health center, and researchers from a local university. Specifically, the team included a bilingual physician, a public health nurse, allied health professionals, a community organizer, a research intern, a Latina social worker, two researchers, and three leaders from the community. Following the CRM, the partnership team engaged in the following steps: (a) reflection of values and health service needs; (b) identification of community and health service needs; (c) brainstorm of ideas and identification of solutions; (d) creation of an action plan and taking action; and (e) contributions to planning sessions for implementing the findings.

(a) **Reflection of values and health service needs**: To identify values and health service needs, the team recommended: conducting a literature review, interviewing leaders from the community of interest, and conducting focus groups. The team organized three focus groups of 90 minutes each through the community health agency. 18 Latino immigrants participated in one of three focus groups.

During the focus groups, participants were asked the following questions:

- What services and things in the community do you value most?
- Why are those services valued?
- What community services do you wish you had that promote your health and well-being, and why?

(b) **Identification of community and health service needs**: Based on the data collected during the focus groups, the literature review, and interviews with community leaders and health professionals about the health needs of Latino immigrants, the partners put together a Concerns Survey.

The survey had two types of questions for each selected issue: one question inquired about the *importance* of the particular issue; the other, about the participant's *satisfaction* with how this issue had been handled in the community. For example, one question asked participants to rate the availability of community programs to prevent or curtail the smoking of cigarettes and tobacco among residents (Table 1.3).

Items rated by participants as high in importance and high in satisfaction are considered *strengths,* while items rated as high in importance and low in satisfaction are considered *needs/concerns*. The 30-item Concerns Survey also included demographic information about participants. With the assistance of the local hospital, health center, and community leaders, 210 individuals completed the survey.

The basic data reported were the mean percentage of importance and the mean percentage of satisfaction for each survey item. The top strengths and problems were listed on a one-page brief report that served as a concise statement of the issues identified by individuals. This is based on the average satisfaction score for all items. Copies of the demographic data were available (Table 1.4). (See expanded data in 12).

(c) **Brainstorming ideas and identifying solutions**. The sponsors arranged a town hall meeting in which Latino immigrants in the community were invited to discuss the dimensions of each issue and to suggest alternatives for preserving the main strengths and for addressing the main concerns identified.

The purpose of the meeting was to provide participants an opportunity to brainstorm solutions to the identified issues and become part of action committees that will work on the community issues of most concern. Those who participated in the focus groups were invited to help plan and assist with the town hall meeting. Several town hall meetings were conducted in the community, the largest attracting about 100 residents. At the town hall meetings the team:

- Introduced all collaborators.
- Obtained a sense of who was in the audience by asking general questions (e.g., how many of you are parents of young children? How many of you are young adults going to school? How many of you work and live in the community?)
- Described the purpose of the meeting: "To understand the dimensions of the issues identified as concerns/needs and discuss ideas for addressing them from their perspective."
- Described briefly the steps already accomplished.
- Shared a one-page summary of main strengths and concerns/needs (celebrate assets, inquire if they agree with the list of strengths, and ask for ways to preserve strengths).

Table 1.3 Sample Question

	How important is to you that …					How satisfied are you that …				
	Not				very	Not				very
… You have access to community programs that prevent/curtail smoking cigarettes and tobacco?	1	2	3	4	5	1	2	3	4	5

Table 1.4 Examples of strengths and concerns for the Latino project included

Community strengths	Community concerns/needs
• Faith-based organizations are available in the community • Support from family and friends is available	• Availability of low-cost dentists who speak Spanish • Availability of programs to help new immigrants • Cigarette and tobacco use prevention programs • Availability of prevention programs to prevent HIV and sexually transmitted disease

- Asked participants to select one concern/need they would like to work on in a smaller group.
  - Provided each group with a flip chart size paper and markers to write down a summary of their discussion.
  - Asked groups to discuss the dimensions of the issues and possible alternative solutions.
  - Discussed the main concerns/needs (items rated high in importance and low in satisfaction). The majority of the town hall meeting discussion should be about the concerns/needs.
- Participants were asked to discuss the following questions in small groups (groups of 10–12):
  - Why is this an issue?
  - How are you and your family affected by the issue?
  - In what circumstances are you affected?
  - What should be done to address the concern/need?
  - What can *you* do to address the concern/need?
  - Discuss specifics about the potential solutions—How? Who? When? What?
- Before wrapping up the meeting, the team obtained a sense of commitment from participants in their willingness to be involved in addressing the issue, and provided an overview of what next steps might be.

(d) **Action planning and action taken.** Provide for open communication of the results. The sponsoring organization disseminated copies of the Concerns Report to all interested parties through active and planned distribution at the town hall meeting. The sponsoring organization had a responsibility to those participating to communicate the findings to the general public and to relevant decision makers (such as agency executives, elected officials, and advisory committees). Several committees with community representation were organized and met for several months to address some of the solutions discussed.

(e) **Contribute to planning sessions for implementing the findings.** Copies of the report were sent to important decision makers that have a say in the concern/need.

(f) **Present the findings when relevant to subsequent decisions**: Concerns Report information has also been used to affect policies such as a new ordinance to extend special needs parking to private property and implementation of enforcement of handicapped parking ordinances. It may also be used to support new procedures such as requirements to inform persons with disabilities of impending changes in public benefits or other relevant decisions. Sponsoring organizations have a responsibility to scan the environment for opportunities to impact such decisions. In this case example, several actions took place including: the development of a resource directory of health services in the community with a section on dentists and other health professionals who offer services in Spanish; implementation of a series of educational workshops about STD and HIV, drug abuse, and cigarette smoking prevention open to the Latino community; and opening of a new health center designed to meet the health needs of the Latino immigrant community.

The team put together a report of the project summarizing the different phases which was distributed to the community, policy makers, health professionals, and the local organizations who sponsored the project.

Conclusion

In this guide, an overview of the NA process illustrating a few strategies that health professionals can utilize was provided. A Needs Assessment process should be used when there is serious intention of acting upon the needs identified by community residents. NA provides a systematic process to gather the opinions, views, and perceptions of those most likely to be impacted by health programs and services. How you gather their views matters as well as what you do with the data. Culturally appropriate and sensitive strategies can provide health professionals, with valuable data to inform programs designed to improve the quality of life of individuals and communities.

References

1. Witkin BR, Altschuld JW. Planning and conducting nees assessment: a practical guide. Thousand Oaks, CA: SAGE Publications; 1995.
2. Tercyak KP, Mays D, DeMarco TA, Sharff ME, Friedman S. Results of an online community needs assessment for psychoeducational interventions among partners of hereditary breast cancer previvors and survivors. J Med Internet Res. 2012;14(1):e15 Epub 2012/01/20.
3. Pregler J, Freund KM, Kleinman M, Phipps MG, Fife RS, Gams B, et al. The heart truth professional education campaign on women and heart disease: needs assessment and evaluation results. J Women's Health. 2009;18(10):1541–7 Epub 2009/09/24.
4. Levy SR, Anderson EE, Issel LM, Willis MA, Dancy BL, Jacobson KM, et al. Using multi-level, multi-source needs assessment data for planning community interventions. Health Promot Pract. 2004;5(1):59–68.
5. Barry MM, Doherty A, Hope A, Sixsmith J, Kelleher CC. A community needs assessment for rural mental health promotion. Health Educcation Res. 2000;15(3):293–304 Epub 2000/09/08.

6. The community tool box—http://ctb.ku.edu/en/default.aspx.
7. Health Services Research Information Central. Community benefit/community health needs assessment. https://www.nlm.nih.gov/hsrinfo/community_benefit.html.
8. Suarez-Balcazar Y, Balcazar F, Taylor-Ritzler T. Using the internet to conduct research with culturally diverse populations: challenges and populations. Cult Divers Ethn Minor Psychol. 2009;15:96–104.
9. Cahill S, Suarez-Balcazar Y. Using photovoice to identify factors that influence children's health. J Allied Health Sci Pract 2012;10(2).
10. Methodologies. Online QDA. http://onlineqda.hud.ac.uk/methodologies.php.
11. Rodriguez L, Suarez-Balcazar Y, Nelson M. Evaluating community-based organizations: implementing an outcomes framework. Chicago: A Self-Directed Guide. Bethel New Life, Inc.; 2001.
12. Suarez-Balcazar Y, Martinez L, Casas-Byots C. A participatory action-research approach to identifying the health needs of hispanic immigrants. Occup Ther Health Care. 2005;19:145–63.
13. Balcazar F, Garcia-Iriarte E, Suarez-Balcazar Y. Participatory action research with colombian immigrants. Hispanic J Behav Sci. 2009;31(1):112–27.
14. Suarez-Balcazar Y, Balcazar F. Functional analysis of concerns in participatory action research. In: Jason L, Glenwick D, editors. Handbook of methodological approaches to community-based research. NY: Oxford, University Press; 2016. pp. 315–323.

Chapter 2
Models of Patient Navigation

Kristen J. Wells and Sumayah Nuhaily

Introduction

Patient navigation is a barrier-focused intervention which aims to assist patients who are completing a healthcare goal [1–3]. Since 1990, patient navigation programs have been widely implemented to help patients obtain timely and high quality healthcare related to cancer and other health conditions. There is evidence that patient navigation is effective in improving receipt of some types of cancer care, including increased rates of cancer screening and diagnostic services [1, 4].

There has been some debate regarding the best methods in designing a patient navigation program and the appropriate training and background of personnel who are responsible for providing patient navigation. Freeman [5], who first coined the term "patient navigation," has suggested because there is a spectrum of various tasks in patient navigation, patient navigators can come from a variety of backgrounds. Some tasks can be accomplished by trained lay patient navigators, whereas other tasks must be performed by professional navigators, such as nurses and social workers [5]. Freeman [6] also suggests that in larger healthcare systems, there should be a system of navigation where multiple patient navigators provide services under the supervision of a navigation coordinator or champion.

Since patient navigation was originally applied to help bring about optimal cancer care, another perspective has suggested that lay navigators be utilized at earlier stages in the cancer continuum (i.e., to provide outreach or facilitate cancer screening), and professional navigators be utilized at the point at which a patient requires cancer diagnostic, treatment, rehabilitation, or survivorship care. For

K.J. Wells (✉) · S. Nuhaily
Department of Psychology, San Diego State University,
6363 Alvarado Court, Suite 103, San Diego, CA 92120-1863, USA
e-mail: kwells@mail.sdsu.edu

S. Nuhaily
e-mail: sumayah.nuhaily@sdsu.edu

E.A. Calhoun and A. Esparza (eds.), *Patient Navigation*,
DOI 10.1007/978-1-4939-6979-1_2

instance, Hopkins and Mumber [7] suggest "optimal providers" at various stages of the cancer continuum by indicating that lay health advisors (trained community volunteers) should provide "outreach navigation," social workers should provide diagnostic navigation, nurses should provide treatment navigation, and nurse practitioners should provide survivorship navigation.

In 2010, the Oncology Nursing Society, the Association of Oncology Social Work, and the National Association of Social Workers issued a Joint Position on the role of oncology nursing and oncology social work in patient navigation [8]. In this position statement, these organizations indicated that nurses and social workers who serve as navigators should provide navigation based on the scope of practice for each discipline and should possess the education and knowledge necessary to perform navigation. This education and knowledge ideally should include "community assessment; cancer program assessment; resolution of system barriers; the cancer continuum; cancer health disparities; cultural competence; and the individualized provision of assistance to patients with cancer, their families, caregivers, and survivors at risk" [8]. The position of the three organizations is that patient outcomes are optimal when a social worker, nurse, and lay patient navigator function as a multidisciplinary team, but that nurses and social workers should supervise and delegate tasks to trained lay navigators or volunteers [8].

On the other hand, others have suggested the most important qualification of a patient navigator is being a "cultural broker and interpreter." In a review of five patient navigation programs designed to assist patients at various stages of the entire cancer continuum, Braun et al. [9] concluded it was important to hire navigators from the communities served by the patient navigation program. Braun and colleagues [9] further specified that a "clinical degree" was not necessary to perform patient navigation, but that effective patient navigators must have certain personal qualities such as being personable; and being willing to: improve the lives of others, provide education to healthcare providers, and advocate for expanded services. In addition, navigators must have the capacity to track services, communicate with professionals, learn about the targeted disease, and refer patients to providers and services [9].

It is clear that there is little consensus regarding the best models for implementing patient navigation. Patient navigation programs are typically designed to meet the needs of a particular community or patient population. However, there is very little information regarding who best fits the profile of someone ideally suited to achieve the desired healthcare outcome targeted by each patient navigation program.

One rich source of information regarding models of patient navigation adopted under various circumstances is the research studies that have been conducted and published in peer-reviewed literature. These studies provide information regarding the background of patient navigators and criteria for selecting patient navigators in addition to providing information regarding the efficacy of the particular patient navigation program for a wide range of health outcomes. A search of PubMed in April 2013 was conducted to find controlled studies of the efficacy of patient navigation for improving a specific health outcome. Excluded were studies where the only outcome was a psychosocial construct, such as knowledge or satisfaction. Since 1995, 49 studies with comparison groups have been conducted to assess the effectiveness of patient navigation in improving cancer care [2, 10–58]. Patient navigation has also been evaluated among patients at risk for cardiovascular disease [59], patients referred for genetic counseling [60] or cardiac rehabilitation [61], as well as patients in need of care for chronic diseases, such as diabetes [62, 63] and human immunodeficiency virus (HIV) [64].

A review of these studies as a whole indicates some trends in the description of patient navigation models. First, there are many studies that provide no or limited information about the personnel who provide patient navigation [11, 17, 20, 24, 29, 32, 43, 51]. In addition, there are several ways in which models of patient navigation have been conceptualized. This is often categorized either by the setting (hospital vs. community) [14, 25, 38], or by the level of education and sometimes type of professional training that the navigator has or has not obtained (lay, college educated, nurse, social worker, case manager, health educator) [10, 13, 15, 19, 21–23, 26–28, 33, 35–42, 44–49, 53–58, 60–64]. Other studies instead only describe a model where the focus is the degree to which the navigator is linguistically or culturally concordant with the community or patient population [2, 12, 16, 18, 30, 31, 50, 52, 59]. Many patient navigation models described in research literature incorporate two or more of these characteristics (e.g., culturally competent lay navigators; professional and lay navigators) [13, 22, 23, 28, 38–40, 42, 44, 45, 47–49, 53, 54, 57, 62, 64]. Chapter 6 "Training Patient Navigators" will go into detail concerning best practices in patient navigation training and key practices for navigators from varied backgrounds.

Prevention

Only one published study, utilizing bilingual patient navigators, evaluated whether patient navigation could improve health behaviors related to cardiovascular disease [59]. The study had mixed findings, as patient navigation was associated with improvements in diet at a twelve-month follow-up, but was not associated with reductions in or cessation of tobacco use [59].

Screening

Twenty-one studies with comparison groups have evaluated whether patient navigation can increase the rates of early detection of disease [11, 13, 15, 17–20, 23, 26, 28, 31–33, 35, 36, 38, 50, 52–55]. To date, all of these studies have focused on the early detection of cancer or precancerous lesions (i.e., cervical cancer screening, colorectal cancer screening). The model of patient navigation was not described well in four studies focused on the early detection of cancer [11, 17, 20, 32].

Although the patient navigation model was not well described, all of these studies found that patient navigation was associated with higher screening rates [11, 17, 20, 32].

One type of navigation model designed to increase cancer screening is patient navigation implemented by lay navigators or community health workers [15, 33, 53, 54]. All of the studies evaluating the efficacy of a lay model found increases in rates of cancer screening associated with patient navigation [15, 33, 53, 54].

There were also a number of studies that had patient navigation models featuring community health educators or health educators [19, 26, 28], nurses or social workers [35, 36], case managers [55], or a combination of a community health worker, a psychology master's degree recipient, and a nursing assistant [23]. Of the three studies investigating the efficacy of patient navigation provided by health educators, all found that screening rates were higher in patients who were provided patient navigation [19, 26, 28]. Of the studies in which navigation was provided by a nurse or social worker, or the combination of a community health worker, a psychology master's degree recipient, and a nursing assistant, all three found that patient navigation was linked with higher rates of screening [23, 35, 36]. The one study which used case managers to provide navigation found patient navigation was associated with obtaining one screening mammogram, but was not necessarily associated with getting mammograms on a regular basis [55].

In five studies, patient navigation models were based on the navigators' racial, cultural, or linguistic similarity to the target population [13, 18, 31, 50, 52]. All five studies found that patient navigation was associated with higher rates of cancer screening [13, 18, 31, 50, 52]. Interestingly, one study compared two different approaches in delivering patient navigation by navigators who were culturally similar to the target population [50]. It found that telephone navigation provided by Native American navigators was more effective than face-to-face navigation provided by Native American navigators [50].

One unique study directly compared "peer" navigators, who were similar to the target population in age, race, and colonoscopy experience, to "professional" navigators, who had experience working with the target population, but were also required to have at least a bachelor's degree [38]. There were no differences found in rates of screening colonoscopy between "peer" and "professional" navigators [38].

Taken together, these studies indicate a range of different patient navigation models have been implemented in studies of the effectiveness of patient navigation in improving cancer screening outcomes. Overall, most studies found that patient navigation was beneficial in improving cancer screening rates, no matter which model was implemented. The one study that compared two patient navigation models found no differences between the "peer" and "professional" navigators in terms of colorectal cancer screening rates. These findings suggest that nearly any model of patient navigation can increase cancer screening. There are no known published studies of the efficacy of patient navigation in improving outcomes related to screening for other diseases.

Diagnosis

Numerous articles described research studies focused on whether patient navigation was effective in increasing the rate of definitive diagnosis following an abnormal cancer screening test or symptom of cancer [29, 30, 45, 47, 49, 57], decreasing the time from a cancer screening abnormality or symptom of cancer to the diagnostic resolution of that abnormality [27, 30, 34, 39, 40, 42–47, 55, 57], completion of a specific diagnostic test [2, 43], or adherence to a recommended follow-up test [48].

Of the studies focused on whether patient navigation improved outcomes related to the receipt of timely cancer diagnostic care, two did not provide information regarding the patient navigation model utilized [29, 43]. Five studies evaluated lay patient navigation programs [27, 42, 44, 46, 47], but there were varying definitions of a "lay" navigator (e.g., completed college education versus high school education; varying experiences in the healthcare system). One study used case managers as navigators [55], whereas a second study used a "healthcare worker" who also happened to be a cancer survivor [34]. Other studies included models of navigation that combined navigators with different levels of training, such as master's-prepared licensed social workers and lay patient navigators [40, 48, 57]; a nurse, dental hygienist, a social worker, and a navigator with a master's degree in business administration paired with community health workers [45]. In addition, three studies indicated that patient navigators were bilingual [2, 30, 39].

Both of the studies that provided very little information on the utilized patient navigation model found patient navigation was associated with improved cancer diagnostic outcomes [29, 43]. One study found that patients who were provided navigation were more likely to receive a biopsy [43] than those who were not provided navigation, and both studies found that patients who received navigation were more likely to receive more timely diagnostic care than those who were not provided navigation [29, 43].

The studies which used a lay patient navigation model had mixed findings [27, 42, 44, 46, 47]. Three studies found that patients who received navigation received diagnostic care faster than those who did not [27, 46, 47], whereas another found no difference in time to diagnosis between those who received navigation and those who did not [42]. A fifth study found that navigation was associated with reduced time from cervical screening abnormality to definitive diagnosis [44]. The same study found that navigation was associated with a significant reduction in the time from breast screening abnormality when diagnostic resolution happened after 60 days, but was not associated with time to diagnostic resolution when the screening abnormality was resolved within 60 days [44]. Another study of a lay navigation model found that the rate of resolution of a screening abnormality was higher in participants who received patient navigation than those who did not [47].

One study used case managers as navigators and found that there were no significant differences in timeliness of follow-up care when care was compared before the navigation intervention compared to after the intervention [55]. Another study utilized a healthcare worker who was also a cancer survivor [34] and found patients who received navigation were provided diagnostic care more quickly than those who were not.

There were several studies which included a combination of different types of navigators from different professional backgrounds. The study that tested an intervention which combined a nurse, a social worker, a dental hygienist, and a navigator with a master's in business administration with community health workers found that patients provided navigation received diagnostic care faster than those who were not provided navigation [45]. In one study which included lay patient navigators and licensed social worker patient navigators, navigation was associated with reduced time from screening abnormality to diagnostic resolution of the abnormality for those whose abnormality resolved after 30 days, but not before 30 days [40]. Other studies that combined a master's-level social worker with a peer counselor found patients provided navigation were more likely to receive diagnostic follow-up and more timely diagnostic care than those who were not provided navigation [48, 57].

There were three studies in which navigation was only defined by the degree to which the navigators were similar to the target population [2, 30, 39]. When navigation was provided by bilingual navigators, it was associated with better adherence to diagnostic follow-up of an abnormal cancer screening test [30], reduced time from an abnormal cancer screening to a definitive diagnosis [39], and completion of a recommended breast biopsy [2].

In one unique study, Native American tribes recruited the patient navigators, some of whom were Native Americans, and some of whom were not. The team of navigators selected by the tribes had various backgrounds, including lay navigators and nurses [49]. The study found that navigation did not help people obtain more timely diagnostic resolution of a screening abnormality when examined 60 or 90 days following the identification of an abnormality, but it did improve the chances of receiving diagnostic resolution by 365 days [49].

When all of the research evaluating the efficacy of patient navigation in improving outcomes related to the diagnosis of cancer is considered, it is clear that most models described in the published studies are associated with improved outcomes. Most of the models that were described were either based on a "lay" model or included several navigators with varying degrees of professional training. There were a few models based on the navigator's competence with or similarity to the target population. There have been no studies evaluating whether patient navigation facilitates the diagnosis of other diseases.

Stage of Cancer at Diagnosis

There were only three studies which evaluated whether patient navigation affected the stage of cancer at diagnosis [14, 25, 51]. In two studies, the navigation model included "community navigators," [14, 25], and there was one study where it was not described [51]. In the study where navigation was described as being performed by "community members", the intervention was not associated with stage of cancer at diagnosis [14]. On the other hand, when navigation was performed by "community health advocates" [25] or was not described [51], it was associated with a statistically significant improved stage of cancer at diagnosis. Given that there is a dearth of studies evaluating the efficacy of patient navigation in improving the stage of diagnosis, little is known regarding the best practices in models of navigation to affect this outcome.

Treatment

Studies have examined whether patient navigation is associated with more timely initiation of treatment following a cancer diagnosis [14, 30, 37, 45, 57, 58]; time of completion of cancer treatment [24, 41]; cancer treatment adherence [22]; cancer treatment interruptions [12, 56]; the degree to which breast cancer treatment quality care indicators were met [10, 16]; and the number of hospitalizations during cancer treatment [21]. However, there were also studies evaluating whether patient navigation improved: symptoms of depression [62]; weight, body mass index, and glycosylated hemoglobin (HbA1c) in patients with diabetes [63]; as well as viral load and adherence to recommended healthcare visits for HIV [64].

There was a large variation in models of patient navigation utilized in studies with treatment-related outcomes. One of the studies did not describe the patient navigation model [24]. One study utilized a lay patient navigator [41], and one study reported that navigation was implemented through a "community member" model [14], with another indicating that navigation was provided by "nonclinical staff" with bachelor's degrees and experiences working with diverse communities affected by HIV [64]. Navigation was provided by a professional navigator in a few studies, including nurses [10, 37, 58], nursing students [63], or by navigators with either a background in social work or nursing [21]. A number of studies had navigation models focused on competence with the target population, either by hiring culturally competent navigators [12], bilingual navigators [30], or bilingual and bicultural navigators [16]. There were several studies that used teams of navigators with multiple professional backgrounds, including one study that combined people with master's degrees in social work with bilingual and bicultural patient navigators [22]; one study which included a nurse, a dental hygienist, a social worker, and a person with a master's degree in business administration plus community health workers [45]; one study which combined a peer counselor and a person with a master's in social work, both of whom had received training in cultural competence [57]; one study that had both hospital-based navigators (nurses) and community research representatives (navigators who live and work in the Native American community of interest) [56]; and one study that reported navigation was provided by "bilingual graduate social work diabetes depression clinical specialists" and "assistant patient navigators" [62].

The study where the navigation model was not fully described found that patient navigation was not helpful in improving time to completion of cancer treatment [24]. The study which utilized the community member model found only modest decreases in the amount of time from diagnosis of cancer to the initiation of cancer treatment [14]. Similarly, in the study which utilized a lay patient navigation model, there were no differences between patients who were provided patient navigation and those who were not in time to completion of primary cancer treatment [41]. On the other hand, navigation provided by "nonclinical staff" with bachelor's degrees was associated with adherence to health care visits and the likeliness of having an undetectable viral load among patients with HIV [64].

With respect to the studies which utilized professional patient navigators alone, there were also mixed findings. In the study where nurses provided navigation, there was an increase in compliance with breast cancer treatment quality care indicators [10]. In contrast, when oncology nurses provided navigation there were no statistically significant reductions in either the time from diagnostic biopsy to consultation with a cancer specialist or initiation of cancer treatment [58]. Similarly, when nursing students provided navigation, there was no improvement in HbA1c, body mass index, or weight among patients with type 2 diabetes [63]. In a study where navigators were required to have a background in nursing or social work, there was no difference between the navigator group and a historical cohort in the total number of days hospitalized, but patients who received navigation had, on average, a mean number of hospitalizations that was lower than those who did not receive navigation [21]. Another study had similar mixed findings in that navigation provided by a nurse was not associated with shortened time to consultation for patients 31–60 years, but was associated with shorter time to consultation among patients older than 60 years [37].

In studies which utilized combined models of patient navigation, the findings were also mixed. In the study which utilized a combined model consisting of "bilingual graduate social work diabetes depression clinical specialists" and "assistant patient navigators," patient navigation was not associated with improvements in depression symptoms [62]. Similarly, a model combining people with master's degrees in social work and bilingual and bicultural patient navigators did not lead to better cancer treatment adherence when compared to enhanced usual care [22]. When a culturally competent peer counselor was paired with a navigator who had a master's degree in social work, there was no difference in the timeliness of initiation of cancer treatment between those who were provided navigation and those who were not [57]. In contrast, when navigation was provided by both nurses and community research representatives, those who received navigation had fewer days of treatment interruptions [56].

The studies which defined navigation models by selecting navigators similar to the target population also yielded mixed results. In a study were the model included culturally competent navigators, patients who were provided navigation had fewer treatment delays than those who were not provided navigation [12]. Similarly, bilingual navigators helped patients initiate cancer treatment faster following a cancer diagnosis [30]. In contrast, while bilingual and bicultural patient navigators helped in general to improve the quality of care as measured by quality indicators during breast cancer treatment and survivorship, there were no statistically significant improvements in individual cancer treatment indicators following the implementation of the patient navigation program, as compared to care given before a patient navigation program was implemented [16].

Taken together, the literature examining the efficacy of patient navigation on improving outcomes related to the treatment of cancer and other diseases has mixed results, regardless of which navigation model was utilized.

Rehabilitation or Survivorship

There are four published controlled studies evaluating whether patient navigation improves care during the period of recovery from a disease [10, 16, 22, 61]. The models that have been researched include a lay patient navigation model [61]; a nurse navigation model [10]; a model which utilized bilingual and bicultural navigators [16]; and a model that included a team of people with master's degrees in social work as well as bilingual and bicultural patient navigators [22]. In a study using a lay patient navigator model, it was found that navigated cardiac patients were more likely to enroll in cardiac rehabilitation than those who did not receive patient navigation [61]. Two studies found that bilingual and bicultural patient navigators [16] and nurse navigators [10] improved the rate of adherence to surveillance mammography among breast cancer survivors. On the other hand, three studies, which each utilized different patient navigation models, found that patient navigation was not effective in improving prescription [10, 16] or receipt [22] of antihormonal medications. There have been so few studies of patient navigation for rehabilitation and survivorship that it is difficult to draw conclusions regarding the efficacy of any particular type of patient navigation model.

Survival

There have also been very few studies of whether patient navigation is related to survival following a cancer diagnosis [14, 51]. One study which evaluated the effect of "community" patient navigators found that patients who received navigation had no better survival rates than those who did not [14], whereas a second study found an increased 5 year survival following implementation of an intervention that included patient navigation [51].

Conclusion

While it is important for patient navigators to be well prepared to provide patient navigation, there is little agreement on which models of patient navigation are best suited to achieve a particular health outcome. There tends to be two considerations in developing patient navigation models. One consideration is competence and familiarity with the target population, which is highlighted by the fact that there is attention to whether the navigation program suits the needs of the target population. The navigators are selected based on their familiarity and competence in working with the target population or their similarity to the target population. The second consideration is whether the professional background of the patient navigator is adequate to perform the duties that he or she is assigned.

The majority of published research has been conducted to evaluate whether various models of patient navigation improve health outcomes related to cancer. Much of the published research has focused on cancer screening and outcomes related to the diagnostic resolution of an abnormal cancer test or symptom of cancer. For the most part, the research indicates that nearly all models, whether defined by professional training or the degree to which the navigator is similar or competent in working with the target population, are effective in improving cancer screening and outcomes related to the diagnostic resolution of a cancer abnormality. On the other hand, it is not clear if patient navigation consistently leads to improved health outcomes in the prevention or treatment of or rehabilitation from a disease, or whether patient navigation affects disease outcomes, such as stage of cancer diagnosis or survival of a disease. Because of the limited number of patient navigation studies related to prevention, survivorship, rehabilitation, morbidity, and survival outcomes, few conclusions can be drawn regarding the best models of patient navigation in these stages of the disease continuum.

Based on the review of the literature, it is surprising how many studies did not describe their navigation model. This may be related to required word limitations in journal articles. Nevertheless, the outcomes observed with models not described tended to mirror the findings of other studies where the models were well described (e.g., navigation was effective in improving care related to screening and diagnosis and mixed with respect to treatment of diseases). Another surprising finding was that, in general, models of patient navigation that focused only on cultural and linguistic competency were successful in improving health outcomes across the continuum of disease. However, this finding is based on the very few studies that have been published.

The findings of the review tend to generally support the ideas of Freeman [5] and, to some extent Hopkins and Mumber [7], who suggest that the degree of professional training should increase either as a disease progresses or as the difficulty of navigation increases. Hopkins and Mumber [7] suggest that lay navigators should only be used for outreach and to increase screening services, but it is clear that lay navigators are often included in models of navigation that are striving to improve diagnostic care and generally have been effective. Sometimes these models only include lay navigators or include lay navigators as part of a team of navigators with different professions, as advocated by the Oncology Nursing Society, the Association of Oncology Social Work, and the National Association of Social Workers [8]. The findings that any model of patient navigation is effective in increasing rates of cancer screening does not support the position of the Oncology Nursing Society, the Association of Oncology Social Work, and the National Association of Social Workers, which states that navigation should ideally be provided by a multidisciplinary team that includes a social worker, nurse, and lay navigator [8]. The multidisciplinary model described by the Oncology Nursing Society, the Association of Oncology Social Work, and the National Association of Social Workers has not consistently been associated with improvements in health care.

Another surprising finding of the review was the relative lack of studies evaluating the efficacy of professional navigator programs where only a professional navigator (nurse or social worker) provided navigation. Most of the studies that included professional navigators used a "combined model" with a mix of professional and lay navigators. Most of the navigation programs that involved nurses were related to improving care for the treatment of disease, which is the area of navigation that has generally had mixed findings with respect to the intervention's efficacy.

A narrative review of published studies has some limitations, including the possibility that studies which find evidence to support patient navigation may be more likely to be published. To date, there has only been one study which compared two models of patient navigation (peer and professional) and which found that the models were similarly effective in helping patients obtain colorectal cancer screening [38]. In the future, this research should be expanded to include more comparative effectiveness and cost-effectiveness studies of patient navigation models.

In conclusion, there is still a lot that is not known about which type of patient navigation model is best suited for a particular situation. To date, nearly all of the published patient navigation research has studied its effectiveness in improving outcomes related to cancer. It appears that nearly any type of model of patient navigation can improve outcomes related to cancer screening. As a disease progresses and requires treatment or rehabilitative care, it is less clear what type of model is best or whether patient navigation is effective at all. Future research is needed to determine the most effective and cost effective patient navigation models.

References

1. Wells KJ, et al. Patient navigation: state of the art or is it science? Cancer. 2008;113(8):1999–2010.
2. Freeman HP, Muth BJ, Kerner JF. Expanding access to cancer screening and clinical follow-up among the medically underserved. Cancer Pract. 1995;3(1):19–30.
3. Dohan D, Schrag D. Using navigators to improve care of underserved patients: current practices and approaches. Cancer. 2005;104(4):848–55.
4. Paskett ED, Harrop JP, Wells KJ. Patient navigation: an update on the state of the science. CA Cancer J Clin. 2011;61(4):237–49.

5. Freeman HP, Rodriguez RL. History and principles of patient navigation. Cancer. 2011;117 (15 Suppl):3539–42.
6. Freeman HP. The origin, evolution, and principles of patient navigation. Cancer Epidemiol Biomarkers Prev. 2012;21(10):1614–7.
7. Hopkins J, Mumber MP. Patient navigation through the cancer care continuum: an overview. J Oncol Pract. 2009;5(4):150–2.
8. Oncology Nursing Society. The association of oncology social work, and the national association of social workers joint position on the role of oncology nursing and oncology social work in patient navigation. Oncol Nurs Forum. 2010;37(3):251–2.
9. Braun KL, et al. Cancer patient navigator tasks across the cancer care continuum. J Health Care Poor Underserved. 2012;23(1):398–413.
10. Weber JJ, et al. Patient navigation and the quality of breast cancer care: an analysis of the breast cancer care quality indicators. Ann Surg Oncol. 2012;19(10):3251–6.
11. Redwood D, et al. The last frontier: innovative efforts to reduce colorectal cancer disparities among the remote Alaska Native population. Gastrointest Endosc. 2012;75(3):474–80.
12. Guadagnolo BA, et al. Patient navigation for American Indians undergoing cancer treatment: utilization and impact on care delivery in a regional healthcare center. Cancer. 2011;117 (12):2754–61.
13. Percac-Lima S, et al. Patient navigation to improve breast cancer screening in Bosnian refugees and immigrants. J Immigr Minor Health. 2012;14(4):727–30.
14. Haideri NA, Moormeier JA. Impact of patient navigation from diagnosis to treatment in an urban safety net breast cancer population. J Cancer. 2011;2:467–73.
15. Lasser KE, et al. Colorectal cancer screening among ethnically diverse, low-income patients: a randomized controlled trial. Arch Intern Med. 2011;171(10):906–12.
16. Chen F, et al. Improving breast cancer quality of care with the use of patient navigators. Am Surg. 2010;76(10):1043–6.
17. Lebwohl B, et al. Effect of a patient navigator program on the volume and quality of colonoscopy. J Clin Gastroenterol. 2011;45(5):e47–53.
18. Phillips CE, et al. Patient navigation to increase mammography screening among inner city women. J Gen Intern Med. 2011;26(2):123–9.
19. Wang X, et al. Evidence-based intervention to reduce access barriers to cervical cancer screening among underserved Chinese American women. J Womens Health (Larchmt). 2010;19(3):463–9.
20. Ma GX, et al. Community-based colorectal cancer intervention in underserved Korean Americans. Cancer Epidemiol. 2009;33(5):381–6.
21. Fillion L, et al. Professional patient navigation in head and neck cancer. Semin Oncol Nurs. 2009;25(3):212–21.
22. Ell K, et al. Cancer treatment adherence among low-income women with breast or gynecologic cancer: a randomized controlled trial of patient navigation. Cancer. 2009;115 (19):4606–15.
23. Lasser KE, et al. A multilevel intervention to promote colorectal cancer screening among community health center patients: results of a pilot study. BMC Fam Pract. 2009;10:37.
24. Schwaderer KA, et al. Evaluation of patient navigation in a community radiation oncology center involved in disparities studies: a time-to-completion-of-treatment study. J Oncol Pract. 2008;4(5):220–4.
25. Gabram SG, et al. Effects of an outreach and internal navigation program on breast cancer diagnosis in an urban cancer center with a large African-American population. Cancer. 2008;113(3):602–7.
26. Christie J, et al. A randomized controlled trial using patient navigation to increase colonoscopy screening among low-income minorities. J Natl Med Assoc. 2008;100(3): 278–84.
27. Ferrante JM, Chen PH, Kim S. The effect of patient navigation on time to diagnosis, anxiety, and satisfaction in urban minority women with abnormal mammograms: a randomized controlled trial. J Urban Health. 2008;85(1):114–24.

28. Fang CY, et al. A multifaceted intervention to increase cervical cancer screening among underserved Korean women. Cancer Epidemiol Biomarkers Prev. 2007;16(6):1298–302.
29. Battaglia TA, et al. Improving follow-up to abnormal breast cancer screening in an urban population. A patient navigation intervention. Cancer. 2007;109(2 Suppl):359–67.
30. Ell K, et al. Patient navigation and case management following an abnormal mammogram: a randomized clinical trial. Prev Med. 2007;44(1):26–33.
31. Nguyen TT, et al. Community-based participatory research increases cervical cancer screening among Vietnamese-Americans. J Health Care Poor Underserved. 2006;17(2 Suppl):31–54.
32. Nash D, et al. Evaluation of an intervention to increase screening colonoscopy in an urban public hospital setting. J Urban Health. 2006;83(2):231–43.
33. Jandorf L, et al. Use of a patient navigator to increase colorectal cancer screening in an urban neighborhood health clinic. J Urban Health. 2005;82(2):216–24.
34. Psooy BJ, et al. Patient navigation: improving timeliness in the diagnosis of breast abnormalities. Can Assoc Radiol J. 2004;55(3):145–50.
35. Weinrich SP, et al. Increasing prostate cancer screening in African American men with peer-educator and client-navigator interventions. J Cancer Educ. 1998;13(4):213–9.
36. Tingen MS, et al. Perceived benefits: a predictor of participation in prostate cancer screening. Cancer Nurs. 1998;21(5):349–57.
37. Basu M, et al. The effect of nurse navigation on timeliness of breast cancer care at an academic comprehensive cancer center. Cancer. 2013;119(14):2524–31.
38. Jandorf L, et al. Implementation of culturally targeted patient navigation system for screening colonoscopy in a direct referral system. Health Educ Res. 2013.
39. Ramirez AG, et al. Navigating latinas with breast screen abnormalities to diagnosis: the Six cities study. Cancer. 2013;119(7):1298–305.
40. Markossian TW, Darnell JS, Calhoun EA. Follow-up and timeliness after an abnormal cancer screening among underserved, urban women in a patient navigation program. Cancer Epidemiol Biomarkers Prev. 2012;21(10):1691–700.
41. Fiscella K, et al. Patient navigation for breast and colorectal cancer treatment: a randomized trial. Cancer Epidemiol Biomarkers Prev. 2012;21(10):1673–81.
42. Wells KJ, et al. A cluster randomized trial evaluating the efficacy of patient navigation in improving quality of diagnostic care for patients with breast or colorectal cancer abnormalities. Cancer Epidemiol Biomarkers Prev. 2012;21(10):1664–72.
43. Hoffman HJ, et al. Patient navigation significantly reduces delays in breast cancer diagnosis in the District of Columbia. Cancer Epidemiol Biomarkers Prev. 2012;21(10):1655–63.
44. Battaglia TA, et al. Boston Patient Navigation Research Program: the impact of navigation on time to diagnostic resolution after abnormal cancer screening. Cancer Epidemiol Biomarkers Prev. 2012;21(10):1645–54.
45. Dudley DJ, et al. Beneficial effects of a combined navigator/promotora approach for Hispanic women diagnosed with breast abnormalities. Cancer Epidemiol Biomarkers Prev. 2012;21(10):1639–44.
46. Raich PC, et al. Patient navigation improves cancer diagnostic resolution: an individually randomized clinical trial in an underserved population. Cancer Epidemiol Biomarkers Prev. 2012;21(10):1629–38.
47. Paskett ED, et al. The Ohio patient navigation research program: does the American Cancer Society patient navigation model improve time to resolution in patients with abnormal screening tests? Cancer Epidemiol Biomarkers Prev. 2012;21(10):1620–8.
48. Ell K, et al. Abnormal cervical screen follow-up among low-income Latinas: project SAFe. J Womens Health Gend Based Med. 2002;11(7):639–51.
49. Warren-Mears V, et al. Impact of patient navigation on cancer diagnostic resolution among Northwest Tribal communities. J Cancer Educ. 2013;28(1):109–18.
50. Dignan MB, et al. A comparison of two native American Navigator formats: face-to-face and telephone. Cancer Control. 2005;12(Suppl 2):28–33.

51. Oluwole SF, et al. Impact of a cancer screening program on breast cancer stage at diagnosis in a medically underserved urban community. J Am Coll Surg. 2003;196(2):180–8.
52. Burhansstipanov L, et al. Breast screening navigator programs within three settings that assist underserved women. J Cancer Educ. 2010;25(2):247–52.
53. Han HR, et al. Tailored lay health worker intervention improves breast cancer screening outcomes in non-adherent Korean-American women. Health Educ Res. 2009;24(2):318–29.
54. Percac-Lima S, et al. A culturally tailored navigator program for colorectal cancer screening in a community health center: a randomized, controlled trial. J Gen Intern Med. 2009;24 (2):211–7.
55. Clark CR, et al. Addressing social determinants of health to improve access to early breast cancer detection: results of the Boston REACH 2010 Breast and Cervical Cancer Coalition Women's Health Demonstration Project. J Womens Health (Larchmt). 2009;18(5):677–90.
56. Petereit DG, et al. Establishing a patient navigator program to reduce cancer disparities in the American Indian communities of Western South Dakota: initial observations and results. Cancer Control. 2008;15(3):254–9.
57. Ell K, et al. Abnormal mammogram follow-up: a pilot study women with low income. Cancer Pract. 2002;10(3):130–8.
58. Koh C, Nelson JM, Cook PF. Evaluation of a patient navigation program. Clin J Oncol Nurs. 2011;15(1):41–8.
59. Shlay JC, et al. Reducing cardiovascular disease risk using patient navigators, Denver, Colorado, 2007–2009. Prev Chronic Dis. 2011;8(6):A143.
60. Rahm AK, et al. Increasing utilization of cancer genetic counseling services using a patient navigator model. J Genet Couns. 2007;16(2):171–7.
61. Scott LB, et al. Effect of patient navigation on enrollment in cardiac rehabilitation. JAMA. Intern Med. 2013;173(3):244–6.
62. Ell K, et al. Depressive symptom deterioration among predominantly Hispanic diabetes patients in safety net care. Psychosomatics. 2012;53(4):347–55.
63. Walker EA, Stevens KA, Persaud S. Promoting diabetes self-management among African Americans: an educational intervention. J Health Care Poor Underserved. 2010;21(3 Suppl):169–86.
64. Bradford JB, Coleman S, Cunningham W. HIV System Navigation: an emerging model to improve HIV care access. AIDS Patient Care STDS. 2007;21(Suppl 1):S49–58.

Chapter 3
Training Patient Navigators for a Reformed Health System

Betsy C. Risendal, Elizabeth M. Whitley, Patricia A. Valverde and Yvonne Kellar-Guenther

Introduction

While PN initially began in the cancer arena, the concept has spread to numerous chronic conditions such as HIV/AIDS, diabetes, cardiovascular disease, asthma/COPD, and mental health [1–4]. Patient navigation is also used in primary care to improve access and care coordination in patient-centered medical homes [5], and The Affordable Care Act calls for PN in the future reformed healthcare system [6]. In 2007, an estimated 120,000 people in the national workforce were performing navigation-related functions in a variety of roles from community workers to members of the healthcare team [7]. Enumeration of the patient navigator workforce is not possible because there is no registry, professional society, or a job code with the Bureau of Labor that encompasses all professions acting in the patient navigator role.

B.C. Risendal (✉)
Department of Community and Behavioral Health, Colorado School of Public Health, 13001 E. 17th Place, Aurora, CO 80045, USA
e-mail: betsy.risendal@ucdenver.edu

E.M. Whitley
Colorado Department of Public Health and Environment, 4300 Cherry Creek Drive South, Denve, CO 80246, USA
e-mail: elizabeth.whitley@state.co.us

P.A. Valverde
Community and Behavioral Health, Colorado School of Public Health, 12477 E. 19th Avenue, T09-141, Buidling 406, M/S B119-406, Aurora 80045, USA
e-mail: patricia.valverde@ucdenver.edu

Y. Kellar-Guenther
Community and Behavioral Health, Colorado School of Public Health, 13001 E. 17th Street, B119, Aurora, CO 80045, USA
e-mail: Yvonne.kellar-guenther@ucdenver.edu

E.A. Calhoun and A. Esparza (eds.), *Patient Navigation*,
DOI 10.1007/978-1-4939-6979-1_3

Patient navigators must have a great deal of knowledge and a bevy of skills, regardless of job title, patient population, disease condition, or practice setting. Building this knowledge and skills base for use in practice is the focus of patient navigator training. However, there is a lack of agreement on what PNs do and what the competencies should be for this emerging workforce [8].

The goal of this chapter is to inform the development and maintenance of effective training programs for patient navigation based on: (1) best practices and common themes from published reports of PN training; (2) rationale and models for competency-based training in PN; (3) strategies for using theory from adult education in PN training methods; (4) practice-based experiences and results from implementation of a large-scale PN training program; and (5) potential models for competency-based training to serve as a practical guide for PN program and training staff, and to encourage a discussion to promote consensus-building and advancement of the field.

(1) ***Best Practices in Patient Navigation Training from Published Literature***

Patient navigation must rely on published reports of training programs to identify best practices in the absence of evidence-based or other standardized methods and curricula. Knowledge of best practices for the training of patient navigators is limited, though the number and type of studies have improved in recent years [9–14]. Below is a summary of findings from these reports.

Content of Training: The training content of published reports varied depending on audience and program, and supports the need for diverse trainings. For example, a key topic covered in lay navigator training programs is navigators' roles and responsibilities. Nurse navigator training is instead centered on three core areas of practice: providing information and education; emotional and supportive care; and facilitation coordination and continuity of care. Relationship building and provision of assistance to patients were also identified as key components to be addressed in all training programs. Topic-specific content, depending on the nature of the navigation program, were also often included such as clinical trials or colorectal cancer guidelines.

Two of the most comprehensive reports of patient navigation training program development and evaluation are provided by Calhoun et al. in 2010 [9] and Klimmek et al. in 2012 [10]. Calhoun et al. describe a standardized training program with the American Cancer Society (ACS), Centers for Medicare and Medicaid Services (CMS), and the Patient Navigator Research Program (PNRP) initiative. Key topics addressed in that program included: background of program/initiative; patient navigator roles and responsibilities; overview of cancer screening and treatment; culture and diversity; communication; introduction to research; and mapping resources and resource management. A subsequent train-the-trainer program based on this initial effort was later conducted by the CMS. The content was refined using the PROCEED Model of Program development, which is sensitive to stakeholder involvement throughout the process. In addition to the above-listed topics, the CMS training added health behavior change, communication in the healthcare team, and CMS eligibility and documentation.

The literature provides support for patient navigation as an evidence-based strategy to reduce barriers to health care most often experienced by underserved patients. These barriers may include cultural beliefs, communication with the healthcare team, and logistical barriers such as transportation and finances. Therefore, more recent articles specific to navigation training indicate the following content, in addition to the skill topics covered in traditional navigator training programs:

- Research ethics including informed consent;
- Orientation to healthcare/healthcare system;
- Motivational interviewing;
- End of life care;
- Legal, regulatory, and insurance issues;
- Healthy behaviors and health belief and behavior theories;
- Identification of barriers at the personal and program level; and
- Program/activity planning.

Navigation trainings for specific programs also often include in-depth training on the disease/condition, such as colorectal cancer or breast cancer screening, or HIV. Thus, best practices from the literature suggest that while content should be tailored to the needs of the audience and program type, a focus on knowledge and skills to address barriers to care is a best practice readily identified in available reports of PN and related training programs.

Methods of Training: Trainings were tailored to the needs and preferences of participants where it is appropriate to take into account culture, education level, health beliefs, and perceived importance of the topics covered. Role playing or "mock" patients or groups, or case scenarios, were often reported as learning activities used during trainings; the use of videos and storytelling was also reported. Use of online or distance modalities was reported in two programs; it was used as pre-work in one training and replaced a full day of training in another. Trainings ranged in length from 6 h to 4 days, with the majority lasting 1–3 days in a workshop format. The number of participants recommended per workshop or training session is not provided in most published reports. The education and experience of the trainers were also not provided by most published reports, making it difficult to identify best practices in terms of trainer qualifications. Maintenance of training was also not detailed. However, it is clear that active engagement of learners in skill-building activities is a common best practice.

Measuring Training Effectiveness: Most programs used some form of program evaluation, though the nature and depth of evaluation activities varied widely from qualitative to quantitative. Importantly, only one study looked at the difference in study outcomes between professional and lay navigators enrolled in the same training program, and found no post-program difference in knowledge and confidence. Validated tools to assess the impact of training are not available in the published literature and few if any authors reported the results of psychometric testing or other measures to assess the validity of these tools. Some form of post-session evaluation including program satisfaction, self-efficacy, and knowledge test was mentioned by most programs. Pretests were offered in relatively few programs. Process evaluation and in-depth interviews were also used to evaluate training programs. Programs reported positive impact, though conclusions as to the efficacy of training are limited due to the wide variety in the nature of the training and the evaluation activities. Initiatives such as the National Institute of Medicine's GEM (Grid-Enabled Measures, www.cancercontrol.cancer.gov/gem) or PROMIS (patient-reported outcomes measurement; www.nihpromis.org) may be important resources in the future to identify peer-reviewed measures and items of use in PN training evaluation as the body of evidence continues to accrue.

(2) ***Competency-based Approach to PN Training***

The development of competency models for various professions is a well-established practice, particularly in healthcare fields such as nursing and pharmacy where standards of performance for licensure or certification have historically been practiced. Common competencies support both individual career growth and programmatic expansion and communication, which are key components in building a strong workforce. Thus, the lack of common PN competencies presents a great challenge in the development of training programs to meet the expectations and needs of the growing number of patient navigators and the populations they serve.

Rationale for Competency-Based Training in PN: The Competency-to-Curriculum Toolkit developed by The Association for Prevention Teaching and Research provides a roadmap for the development of effective training and education for the public health workforce, where there is often a lack of defined competencies similar to PN [11]. In this Toolkit, the authors' state that identifying learners by audience type or profession (e.g., nurse, community health worker) or program area (e.g., tuberculosis, cancer, maternal health) may have advantages in the short term, but lacks the needed depth to ensure long-term gains in the establishment of an emerging profession. Instead, a training program focused on competencies helps to assure individuals will be well prepared to conduct their job duties in real-world settings. Further, competency-focused approaches facilitate multidisciplinary teams and programs working together effectively to address cross-cutting, complex problems often encountered in health and health care. Competency training is related to but distinct from other forms of workplace trainings and documentation such as job descriptions, performance reviews, self-assessments, or employee orientation sessions.

Competency has been defined as, "…a combination of knowledge, skills and performance that results in the ability to apply knowledge, skills and judgment in practice" [12]. The previously described standardized patient navigator training program (ACS, CMS, PNRP) utilized a performance checklist as a first step toward an accepted definition of competencies for navigators [9]. This checklist centered on four broad areas of competency: client interaction, case management, intervention, and documentation. Tasks were specified within each of these areas. For example, client interaction tasks focused around clarity of explanation of the program and purpose and understanding patient needs. Case management covers assessment of patient barriers to care, and developing an assistance plan with follow-up. Intervention tasks center around provision of educational and other resources; and documentation covers accurate and complete entry of activities into program records.

Core competencies for navigators have also been proposed by the National Coalition of Oncology Nurse Navigators [13]. Similar to the above, the role of the nurse navigator is conceptualized to include health education, health promotion, care coordination, counselor, research coordinator, and patient advocate. Other agencies and institutions (e.g., C-Change, Pfizer) have published patient navigation toolkits to move the field toward a common definition of patient navigation including roles and responsibilities, although a commonly accepted set of competencies for patient navigation has yet to be reached.

Several existing professions closely related to patient navigation have known competency sets for various levels of worker which are generally utilized for certification at either the state, national, or international level. These include Public Health practitioners; Sexually Transmitted Disease/Human Immunodeficiency Virus (STD/HIV) Counselor; Health Education Specialist (CHES); and Community Health Workers (CHWs). Similar to the field of patient navigation, several have attempted to enumerate competencies for the CHW workforce, which has proven difficult due to the variety of roles. However, Texas, Ohio, and Minnesota have required certification of CHWs to cover services. Additionally, Indiana and Alaska allows payment for CHWs only within programs that provide standardized training [7, 15, 16]. Core competencies for CHWs in the state of Texas are listed as an exemplar, although CHWs typically operate at the beginning (or opposite end) of the care continuum from patient navigators: interpersonal skills, capacity building skills, service coordination skills, teaching skills, and knowledge base.

Potential Competency-based Model for PN Training and Implications in Workforce Development: The practice of psychology organizes competencies using a three-dimensional model comprised of integrally related (1) foundational, (2) functional, and (3) developmental competencies [17]. Foundational competencies are comprised of the knowledge, attitudes, and values essential to performance of the functional competencies. Functional competencies are methods and skills necessary for performance of key tasks. Developmental competencies are effective integration of foundational and functional competencies and continued professional growth. Use of this model facilitates not only standardization of performance but also assessments of performance. Competencies put forth by the national standardized training program previously described fit well with this three-dimensional model, as follows:

Foundational Competencies—Demonstrate Knowledge and Awareness

Domain: Ethical, legal, and professional issues

Competency: Demonstrates professionalism through adherence to organizational rules and regulations, ethical principles, and boundaries of the navigator's scope of work.

Examples of Performance Behaviors

- Implements the navigator scope of work and role within the healthcare team.
- Supports patient/clients' rights in health decision-making.
- Maintains patient/client confidentiality.
- Adheres to basic policy and procedures in the health care and employer environment.
- Adheres to legal standards relevant to performance of job duties such as reporting of abuse/neglect or behavior that is imminently harmful to self or others.
- Preserves human subject protection.
- Identifies and explains patient/client rights and responsibilities.
- Consults with other members of the healthcare team on patient/client concerns that fall outside his/her scope of work.
- Maintains appropriate and accurate documentation of work performed.
- Maintains appropriate personal boundaries with health staff and clients/patient/clients and family.
- Acts within scope of work.

Domain: Health beliefs and behavior

Competency: Understands the impact of individual health beliefs and behavior on healthcare decisions.

Examples of Performance Behaviors

- Identifies individual and cultural diversity in views of wellness/illness and disability.
- Demonstrates effective strategies for delivering health information.
- Recognizes stages of behavior change.
- Understands motivators for behavior change.
- Integrates motivators for behavior change and the role of familial/social and environmental factors in designing effective treatment strategies.

Domain: Psychology of illness

Competency: Integrates knowledge of the social and emotional aspects of health into patient/client, caregiver and family interactions and support.

Examples of Performance Behaviors

- Applies understanding of common reactions to a chronic disease diagnosis and living with chronic disease in communications with patient/clients, caregivers, and family members.
- Recognizes common signs and symptoms of pathological reactions and/or mental illness and discusses them with other members of the health team.
- Acknowledges implications of psychological factors on how patient/clients, caregivers, and family members are able to effectively work with the patient/client navigator.
- Recognizes issues in death and dying and their impact on relationships between patient/clients, caregivers, and family members.

Domain: Disease-specific knowledge
Competency: Demonstrates basic knowledge of health promotion, disease prevention, and common disease care continuums.

Examples of Performance Behaviors

- Understands basic pathophysiology of common chronic diseases.
- Provides basic health information relevant to screening—diagnosis—treatment of chronic diseases to patient/clients, caregivers, and family members.
- Identifies emerging evidence and impact on practice.
- Recognizes common signs and symptoms of health emergencies and acts accordingly.
- Acknowledges common biopsychosocial impact of health procedures on patient/client, caregivers, and family members.
- Demonstrates knowledge of and adherence to infection control, medical documentation, and medical records procedures.

Domain: Healthcare system structure and function
Competency: Apply understanding of the healthcare system to improve client/patient/client care.

Examples of Performance Behaviors

- Understands the role of each member of the healthcare team and their required skills and competencies.
- Utilizes the knowledge of public and private insurance/payor programs, economic issues in the healthcare setting to make appropriate referrals to payor programs.
- Demonstrates knowledge of healthcare specialty disciplines.
- Demonstrates understanding of multiple specialties within care teams.
- Maintains appropriate recordkeeping and charting to facilitate coordinated care.

Domain: Resource and referral mechanisms and sources
Competency: Identifies and utilizes resources and appropriate referrals to reduce patient/client barriers to care.

Examples of Performance Behaviors

- Identifies local, state, and federal assistance programs and informational resources relevant to patient/client's care.
- Conducts professional networking with other patient/client navigators to enhance knowledge of resources.
- Documents referrals made on behalf of patient/client.
- Maintains relationships with referral sources.
- Effectively advocates for appropriate community and social service resources for patient/clients.

Functional Competencies—Demonstrate Skill and Understanding of Process

Domain: Patient/client/Client assessment

Competency: Conducts effective patient/client/client interviews to identify needs and strengths of patient/client/client.

Examples of Performance Behaviors

- Identifies personal and system barriers to patient/client's use of the health system.
- Identifies patient/client and family strengths for managing the patient/client's current health condition.
- Elicits and recognizes common risk factors for other physical and emotional conditions.
- Establishes effective client relationships by building trust and open communication
- Provides continuous monitoring and follow-up to ensure that the client assessment is relevant to the current situation and makes changes to the care plan accordingly.

Domain: Client Interaction and Communication Skills

Competency: Establishes a professional relationship with patient/client/family by building trust and communicating in a collaborative manner.

Examples of Performance Behaviors

- Engages client in preferred language.
- Uses active and reflective listening techniques.
- Identifies health communication issues such as health literacy that affect client knowledge and attitudes about their health care.
- Adapts oral and written communication skills to patient/client's literacy level.
- Demonstrates professional conduct and attitude.

Domain: Work within health patient/client care team and community
Competency: Demonstrates collaboration within and across the care team, patient/client, and community agencies.
Examples of Performance Behaviors

- Proactively anticipates barriers and challenges for patient/client in using healthcare and communicates these to the healthcare team.
- Adheres to the health care recommendations provided by the health team.
- Participates in the development of effective care strategies as part of an interdisciplinary client care team.
- Establishes relationships with local community leaders and communicates relevant program information.

Domain: Healthcare team-patient/client communication
Competency: Assists in the development and enhancement of appropriate and open communication between the patient/client and the healthcare team.
Examples of Performance Behaviors

- Assists client in identifying concerns and questions to share with healthcare team.
- Reiterates provider recommendations using language that is clear to the patient/client.
- Participating in the development of effective treatment strategies as part of an interdisciplinary care team.
- Provides cultural mediation as needed, acting as a liaison between the healthcare system and client.
- Engages client in preferred language and/or obtains an interpreter as needed.
- Utilizes communication techniques that foster mutual respect.

Domain: Appropriate referral for behavioral health or emergency medical care
Competency: Arranges referrals to behavioral and physical health providers for additional professional support.
Examples of Performance Behaviors

- Recognizes and acts upon signs and symptoms of serious behavioral or physical health conditions, by addressing these with the client and healthcare team.
- Assists in the referral process and conducts timely follow-up.
- Communicates with client and healthcare team to facilitate palliative care as appropriate.

Domain: Care Coordination
Competency: Accesses, evaluates, and uses appropriate information and resources in designing client/patient/client-centered care plans.

Examples of Performance Behaviors

- Assesses client needs, strengths, and readiness for change.
- Engages the patient/client in problem solving to identify, prioritize, and reduce barriers to care.
- Performs collaborative goal setting with patient/client and healthcare team.
- Facilitates patient/client knowledge and skills for managing their health.
- Conducts appropriate and timely referrals to clinical and professional staff.
- Integrates care strategies with patient/clients' personal and cultural values.
- Creates and implements a patient/client-centered plan of care, integrating clients' personal and cultural values.
- Identifies individualized process and outcome measures for monitoring client progress and providing appropriate feedback to patient/client.
- Monitors client progress through ongoing follow-up.

Domain: Client activation, education, and support
Competency: Facilitates the engagement of the patient/client in their health.
Examples of Performance Behaviors

- Appropriately identifies the informational needs of the client and family.
- Evaluates and selects educational materials that match the health literacy level and cultural and linguistic needs of the patient/client.
- Provides interpretation of educational materials.
- Supports the client's ongoing need for information at different times throughout the episode of care.
- Utilizes effective techniques to empower personal actions relevant to adherence to health recommendations.
- Encourages health promotion and disease prevention behaviors to maximize health potential.
- Conducts referral to community resources and stimulation of clients' health promotion and disease prevention behaviors.

Developmental Competency—Display Integrative Capacity of All Knowledge and Skills

Domain: Professionalism and development
Competency: Optimizes practice as patient/client navigator through continual professional development.
Examples of Performance Behaviors

- Recognizes one's limitations in health knowledge and professional competencies.
- Adopts healthy work practices to avoid burn-out.

- Identifies need for supervision and support.
- Demonstrates a commitment to self-assessment.
- Seeks out continuous learning and improvement in performance.

Domain: System change

Competency: Seeks to improve systems of care for patient/clients through the identification of systemic barriers and challenges.

Examples of Performance Behaviors

- Identifies which barriers may be systemic.
- Generates possible solutions with the client, healthcare team, and organizational leadership.
- Communicates solutions with organizational leadership to eliminate these systemic barriers.

Domain: Program development and management

Competencies: Participates in patient/client navigator program development, improvement, and evaluation.

Examples of Performance Behaviors

- Demonstrates the capacity to develop an effective navigator program.
- Develops program policies and procedures utilizing evidence-based and research-driven methods.
- Establishes effective referral networks with community-based agencies, other providers and patient/client navigators.
- Fosters relationships with community leaders, particularly within communities served.
- Develops program evaluation components which include process and outcomes indicators.
- Implements and monitor process and outcome measures.
- Reports evaluation results to funders and institutional leaders.
- Communicates evaluation results to peers in the research and navigator community through publications or presentations.

Using these foundational, functional, and developmental competencies informed by National Cancer Institute Patient Navigation Research Program (NCI PNRP), program managers at the American Cancer Society (ACS), Center for Medicare and Medicaid Services (CMS), and the authors represents the beginning of integration of competency from training into practice. Supervised work followed by certification upon demonstration of the core competencies can serve to provide employers with the confidence needed of a competent workforce.

(3) ***Strategies for Adult Learning Theory in PN Training***

Best practices from the PN training literature described previously suggest that role playing, scenarios, storytelling, and other methods of active learning engagement were present in most if not all published reports. Active engagement is one of the recognized methods for adult learners, and application of theories of adult learning can further inform the approach to PN training. The theory of andragogy (adult learning) as described by Knowles et al. in 1998 indicates:

1. Adults need to know why they are learning something.
2. Adults learn through doing.
3. Adults are problem-solvers.
4. Adults learn best when the subject is of immediate use.

These principles can be illustrated using various strategies in the training of adult learners. The participants need to know why they should learn something new and see the relevancy; learners should be encouraged to be self-directed; adults bring life experiences and a sense of who they are to the classroom which can be integrated to enrich the learning experience; students should see the benefits of the instruction to coping with their daily life and work tasks; and adult learners must be motivated to learn, and this motivation is likely different for each student (typical motivators include job satisfaction, increased self-esteem, improved quality of life) [17].

Competency-based training for PNs lends itself well to application of the above-described approaches. For example, many PNs who represent the potential workforce have valuable life experiences from their previous professional positions or key relationships with communities. These life experiences can be built into case studies or useful examples in role playing or other training activities. Working toward a certification or other means of recognition of competency provides a motivation for career growth and recognition of navigators as important members of the healthcare team. This can be emphasized in trainings by facilitated discussions with sharing of job descriptions and organizational charts to discern job roles and potential avenues for collaboration and communication. Focusing on skill acquisition relevant to reducing barriers to care will help PNs to see benefits of the training in their daily work and identify ways to improve patient outcomes through their activities. For example, simulated case studies can aid PNs in anticipating common barriers and selecting appropriate strategies to address them, using appropriate examples from practice. These adult-learning based approaches, in contrast to traditional didactic learning methods common to professional trainings, highlight opportunities to inform the development of PN training that is both effective and engaging to the target audience.

(4) ***Practice-based Example of PN Training Program Development and Implementation: The Patient Navigator Training Collaborative (PNTC)***

Available evidence from a review of the PN training literature indicates that most patient navigation programs are developing in-house trainings to meet their unique program needs, or otherwise supplementing the few outside programs available that may be expensive or too general to be entirely useful. However, few examples from the literature are available to describe the development, implementation, and evaluation of an ongoing PN training effort. This information is needed by both program developers and practitioners in order to identify best practices and methods to ultimately sustain PN programs and associated necessary training for implementation. The PNTC is provided here as an example of how PN training was approached by a group of key stakeholders, how implementation strategies were deployed, and describes the impact and efficacy of training for this target population. Further, the evaluation program for the PNTC is provided as an example to stimulate other programs to collect their own high-quality data to support quality improvement and training program maintenance efforts.

PNTC Background and Approach to Training Program Development: The purpose of the PNTC is to provide high-quality training to meet the need of a growing PN workforce in Colorado. This includes training new patient navigators and providing supplemental training opportunities for those currently serving in the patient navigator role. Secondary to meeting this immediate need, the goal is to establish a presence in the field of navigation to facilitate networking and serve as a resource in the national discussion.

Funding for program development was provided by state initiative through competitive grant applications to the Colorado Cancer, Cardiovascular Disease, and Chronic Pulmonary Disease Prevention, Early Detection, and Treatment Program, or CCPD grants program. Funding was initially obtained for the 2006–2009 period, and then reinstated in 2012 following a hiatus due to state budget issues. While not all PN programs will have the capability to obtain this kind of resource infrastructure, recognition of the need for initial input of resources by policy makers and institutional leadership is key to the long-term success of a PN training program. The PNTC was funded based on the rationale that standardization of training would not only facilitate implementation but evaluation of the impact of the growing PN workforce in Colorado.

It is well-established that the patient, provider, and system level barriers addressed by the PN workforce are multifaceted and cross-cutting. Therefore, the composition of PNTC membership is synergistically comprised of a multidisciplinary and multi-institutional group representing the fields of nursing, community health work, psychology, palliative care, communication, social work, epidemiology, and public health. Supervisors of PN programs were also intentionally included to ensure that training activities were relevant to job responsibilities. This structure serves as an example of the commitment and resources needed to develop a PN training program. In keeping with the previously described Competency—to-Curricula Toolkit, one of the first tasks of the PNTC was to define the target audience (see Fig. 3.1). While this PN model may or may not have direct applicability to all programs or settings, the development of a model to describe the target audience and tasks for the training is an essential component of a well thought-out approach.

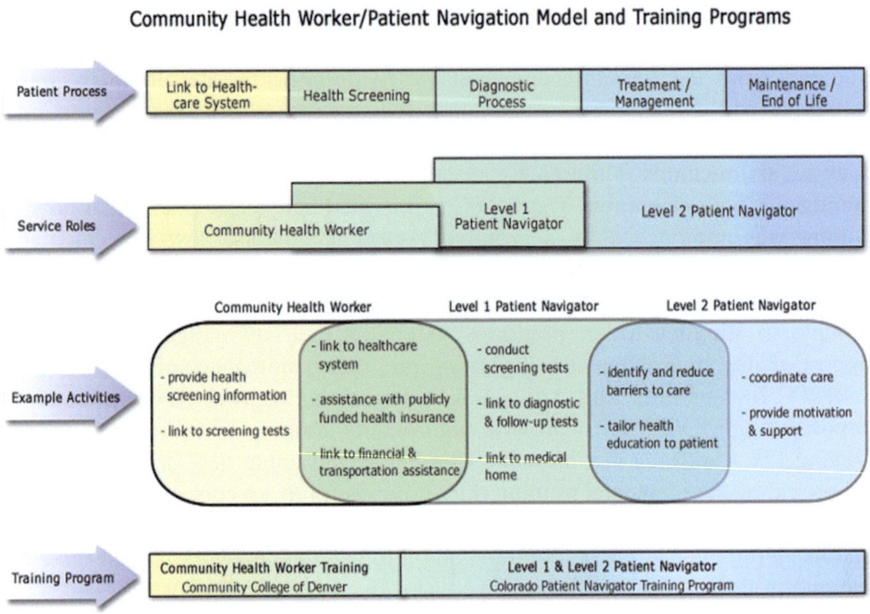

Fig. 3.1 Community Health Worker/Patient Navigation Model and Training Programs

Points of differentiation between Level 1 and Level 2 patient navigators include the intensity of the care coordination, the time spent on individual client needs and length of relationship. Level 1 navigators have shorter relationships with their clients and navigate them to specific types of care and services. Level 2 navigators may have much longer relationships, patients with more in-depth needs, navigate the client to multiple types of care and resources, and work with multiple service providers on behalf of the client. The knowledge and skills are basic for Level 1 and more advanced for Level 2.

In the absence of PN-specific recognized standards or guidelines, members of the PNTC engaged at the start of the project in 2006 in a deliberative process which resulted in the following nine themes for the content of the training program: History, purpose, and role of patient navigators; patient communication and assessment skills; health communication and health literacy; resources in patient navigation; physical aspects of chronic disease; psychosocial aspects of chronic disease; professional boundaries in patient navigation; ethics and decision-making; and end-of-life issues. Notably, these topics are similar to those now reported in the literature as best practices, described previously.

PNTC Training Program Implementation Strategies and Results: Content was offered in modules to offer flexibility to participants. Content-oriented teams were assigned based on the members' expertise to identify competencies and then objectives, along with the corresponding content for each theme. This intentional process of course development that is driven by competencies is critical to training program development principles. Periodic meetings were held for the content teams to present their material and receive feedback from other team members, which also promoted synergy in content and delivery of material. The results of each team's efforts were translated into Facilitator Guides to document the content and method of delivery related to each objective, also identified as a best practice in the literature.

Wherever possible, educational objectives were taught by facilitated learning methods using adult learning theory strategies. Skill-building objectives were taught in role-plays (diads and triads), demonstrations, videos, and case scenarios where participant skills could be observed. Some members of educational teams received a two-day training in how to conduct interactive training classes and facilitate discussions; others had experience in adult education. Ongoing evaluation activities (see below) by peer facilitators identified the strong need for co-facilitation during course delivery to ensure that workshops were structured to include important elements of group learning such as: establishment of class "rules" by participants; use of a "parking lot" for off-topic issues raised during discussions; observation of small groups during class exercises; and note-taking/summarizing for participants.

As of October 2012, PNTC has trained 645 individuals in Level I basics of patient navigation with the above-described format through in-person workshops; 493 of these or 76%, worked in Colorado. Thirty-three participants completed the 6-week, instructor-led synchronous Level II training on "Psychosocial Aspects of Chronic Disease."

The PNTC has also delivered online courses using self-paced tutorials and instructor-led, synchronous trainings to meet the distance-learning needs of rural or geographically distance programs. Between 2009–2010, 1449 participants completed the introductory self-paced tutorial titled, "Patient Navigation and the Healthcare System." In the same period, 692 participants completed the Level 2 self-paced tutorial titled, "Introduction to Chronic Disease: Impact and Risk Factors". Importantly, the enrollment in these tutorials further increased in 2011, with an additional 1203 completing the introductory tutorial and 451 completing the second tutorial. This represents a nearly 30% increase in annual enrollment between 2010 and 2011, demonstrating continued interest and need.

PNTC Program Evaluation Plan and Outcomes: In order to evaluate the assumptions about the target audience used for course development and continuous improvement, the training evaluation surveys collected respondent characteristics—a key activity of any training program evaluation. Of the 645 trained in the Level I basics: 7% had a high school or GED, 17% had some college, 15% had an associates or technical degree, 33% had bachelors and 20% had a masters or Ph.D.

The range in participant backgrounds included: healthcare providers (20–22%); lay people (20–46%); paraprofessionals such as nurse or health educators (5–20%); and social workers/counselors (5–6%). Workplace setting/funding sources for these navigators included healthcare systems (11–57%); community agency (1–24%); and other foundation or organization (1–21%). An additional 1–52% said they were volunteers without pay. Disease-related issues handled by navigators trained by the

PNTC include breast, cervical, and colorectal cancer; diabetes; cardiovascular disease, asthma/COPD; mental health. Finally, the navigation experience has ranged dramatically between students. While some trainees are new to the field, less than 6 months, (range 10–60% across all training environments) others have been navigators for over 5 years (24–55% across all training environments). The mix of experience and educational backgrounds has proven to be a challenge in implementation of the training program, as reflected by the range in respondent scores when asked, "I learned something new." Taken in sum, these results support the need for PN training that can meet the needs of a heterogeneous workforce with incremental increases in responsibility. More recently, PNTC has trained a specific group of volunteer patient navigators called "Boomers". These Boomer volunteers are mid-career, experienced community members. The influx of these participants highlights the need for training programs that can be quickly tailored as PN initiatives continue to increase in a variety of settings, and suggests that PN training programs must plan for this flexibility during development.

In the absence of a credentialing body/program, PNTC has relied on participant feedback to refine and identify gaps in the curriculum. Thus, evaluation data is a critical component of any PN program to both provide evidence of impact and facilitate continuous improvement. The outcomes of the evaluation have focused primarily on changes in knowledge and satisfaction with the training. After each training, the evaluation data is reviewed by the team; the team discusses what changes need to be made to the existing curriculum and what new topics need to be added to better meet course objectives. Through this process the PNTC training has expanded from a 2-day to 4-day Level 1 training. Thus, resources for program adaptation should be anticipated throughout PN program implementation.

Overall, the perceived impact of the training program to date has been high. To measure impact, pre and post knowledge tests were administered in 2008, 2009, and 2011. In 2011, 71% of the participants had increases in posttest knowledge scores but there were still 22% whose scores stayed the same, highlighting the need for trainings that can apply to a workforce with varied backgrounds and experience. The evaluation forms also collect participant satisfaction/perceived utility, assessed via self-report with a 15-item survey which uses constructs from the training transfer literature on a five-point scale [18]. When asked, "The quality of the program content met my expectations and was current, evidence-based", responses were similarly high and ranged from 4.0 to 4.9. The average participant overall satisfaction score is 4.0. This type of evaluation, based on training literature, represents an important construct to include in PN training program evaluation plans.

(5) ***Key Practices from Relevant Competency-based Training Models***: Patient navigators typically come from a variety of backgrounds with different education levels, ranging from a High School diploma or equivalency to the Master's level. In some cases, such as nursing and social work, an advanced college degree and licensure is required to practice. However, patient navigation is also increasingly viewed as a position on the career ladder for lay health workers who often have less formal education, yet more experience with the

patient groups which may benefit most from PN. This group of patient navigators may be (1) racially or ethnically concordant with the community served by the navigator program, or (2) survivors, former or current patients. College education and training are not typically required for entry level community health workers, but established relationships with the community and patient population are key requirements. Another group of patient navigator students are the healthcare professionals from other countries who are not licensed to practice in the United States.

In the absence of a consensus set of qualifications, core competencies, or national standards, looking to other fields that teach to core competencies with analogous components to the above-described characteristics of the potential PN workforce may provide useful insights. More specifically, models that train a heterogeneous workforce and allow for incremental responsibility as skills and expertise increase can address two notable features of PN. Two such models are tobacco treatment specialists and substance abuse addiction counselors, as described below.

Tobacco Treatment Specialists (TTS) are individuals who have completed a training taught to a consensus set of core competencies. In addition, certification is provided after completion of a required amount of hours and demonstration of the integration of core skills. The certification process and core competencies are maintained by a national association with an interdisciplinary board. With the certification, employers and healthcare systems are ensured that the individual is competent in the most evidence-based strategies of supporting tobacco cessation both individually or group, in-person or via the phone and regardless of whether the person is a nurse, social worker or lay. TTS is an example of a core set of competencies that all trainees can acquire and implement within their current work or as a sole job function.

Another example of a training model with incremental skills, competencies, and respective certification is addiction counseling training. There are a myriad of options related to working in addictions counseling from Level 1 counselor with a high school diploma up to master's level licensing. The employer can determine which level is required for the position given the job duties and client mix. Although the states may vary in educational and supervised work experience, there is a career ladder within the field starting with high school level certification through master's and doctorate level licensure. The requirements are long term (i.e., 6000 hours supervised experienced with 270 contact hours) and the educational credit can lead to a baccalaureate degree, providing a career pathway to those beginning as trained lay counselors.

Both models share four key practices

(1). Lay, professional and bachelor's level prepared individuals have potential employment in the field.
(2). A national set of consensus core competencies implemented regionally or at state level.
(3). Core competencies based on evidence-based practice and the ability to update training with new scientific results that impact the field.

(4). Substantial supervised work to ensure the integration of competencies into practice.

In the field of patient navigation, the workforce is made up of both professional and lay (nonprofessional) patient navigators. PN training programs must develop strategies to cope with the heterogeneous level of experience, skills, and educational levels of navigators seeking skill development and enhancement, similar to these two models. In Dr. Freeman's recent article on the principles of patient navigation, he acknowledges and supports the notion that individuals with varying educational backgrounds can provide patient navigation [19]. In fact, Dr. Freeman outlines the concept of varying levels of skills and expertise that are appropriate at different points of time during the disease/health continuum to further provide guidance for program implementation. However, recognized competencies to guide training for each of these heterogeneous levels and/or timepoints have yet to be established for PN.

One question to answer is whether there are models for guidance on the establishment of patient navigators as members of the healthcare team? Training programs need to tie their content back to these competencies to ensure some consistency in navigator training programs as well as consistency in the field once navigators begin their work. In addition to educational preparation and communication, examples of other questions to be answered in terms of implementation of standardized training program for patient navigators include:

- Maintenance training: Can all competencies be achieved in a one-time training program, or is maintenance or booster training required to maintain a level of competence? What type of continuing education should be provided?
- Competency assessment: How will developmental competencies be assessed? Should patient navigators be required to perform a practicum to demonstrate competency or can video data obtained during training role-plays be used to assess competencies? Should observation and supervision be an important component of this assessment?

While tying training content to the competencies is important, there are nuances that can be missed. Communication skills, both written and spoken, are essential to successful performance of patient navigator job duties within the complex health system. At the same time, hiring and training bilingual staff with the skills to communicate effectively with disparate populations in a multilingual environment requires both flexibility in training and employment. After conducting hundreds of interviews with patient navigator programs, the Institute of Alternative Futures concluded in their 2007 report that the first responsibility of patient navigators is to, "Facilitate communication among patients, family members, survivors and healthcare providers, and coordinate care among providers." Further, they describe an effective navigator as:

- Compassionate, sensitive, culturally attuned to the people and community being served and able to communicate effectively.

- Knowledgeable about the environment and healthcare system.
- Connected with critical decision makers inside the system, especially financial decision makers." [20]

The patient navigation fields needs to think through how these nuances can be captured in the competencies listed and how to ensure that navigators receive appropriate training and support for these activities. The current state of implementation of practice, as well as the state of the science, indicates that a call to action for the development of competency-based, standardized training for patient navigators is needed. The route to get there has many possible paths but should include:

- Enumeration of patient navigators in the workforce;
- Gathering of job analysis data to work toward a common definition of roles and responsibilities that can inform relevant competency-based standards;
- Assessment of desired training on part of key stakeholders including employers and clients of patient navigators;
- Funding of projects to collect evaluation data using consistent metrics and including cost as an outcome;
- Formalization of "hand-offs" or care transfers in the medical system that can be assisted with patient navigation programs to improve patient outcomes, and skill development in this area;
- Integration of best practices in adult education into existing and planned program-specific training programs for patient navigators;
- Utilization of recognized pedagogical principles in the development and implementation of curricula, including the development of objectives driven by desired competencies and target audience needs;
- Follow-up of training participants to study the transfer and maintenance of knowledge and skills from training programs;
- Evaluation of the pros and cons of certification based on competencies using other related fields as a guide.

These kinds of competency-driven approaches to training require continued involvement of policy makers, advocates, educators and the workforce to identify needed knowledge and skills that can be applied to real-world settings in order to ensure that patient navigation fulfills the promise offered by healthcare reform.

References

1. Van Walleghem N, Macdonald CA, Dean HJ. Evaluation of a systems navigator model for transition from pediatric to adult care for young adults with type 1 diabetes. Diabetes Care. 2008;8:1529–30 Epub 2008 May 5.
2. Bradford JB, Coleman S, Cunningham W. HIV System Navigation: an emerging model to improve HIV care access. AIDS Patient Care STDS. 2007;21(Suppl 1):S49–58.

3. Manderson B, Mcmurray J. Navigation roles support chronically ill older adults through healthcare transitions: a systematic review of the literature. Health Soc Care Community. 2012;20(2):113–27.
4. Paskett ED, Harrop P, Wells KJ. Patient navigation: an update on the state of the science. CA Cancer J Clin. 2011;61(4):237–49.
5. Ferrante JM, Cohen DJ, Crosson JC. Translating the patient navigator approach to meet the needs of primary care. J Am Board Fam Med. 2010; 23(6):736-44. PubMed PMID: 21057069.
6. Public Law 111–148. Patient protection and affordable care act of 2010. Washington, DC.
7. Community Health Worker National Workforce Study. Health research services administration, Washington, DC, 2007.
8. Wells KJ, Battaglia TA, Dudley DJ, et al. Patient Navigation: state of the art or is it science? Cancer. 2008;113(8):1999–2010.
9. Calhoun EA, Whitley EM, Esparza A, et al. A national patient navigator training program. Health Promot Pract. 2010;11(2):205–15.
10. Klimmek RK, Noyes E, Edington-Saunders K, Logue C, Jones R. Wenzel training of community health workers to deliver cancer patient navigation to African American seniors. J. Prog Community Health Partnersh. 2012;6(2):167–74. doi:10.1353/cpr.2012.
11. http://www.phf.org/resourcestools/Documents/Competency_to_Curriculum_Toolkit08.pdf www.asph.org/competency-to-curriculum-toolkit08; accessed on 6/25/2013.
12. Sanford B, editor. Strategies for maintaining professional competence: a manual for professional associations and faculty. Toronto, Canada: Canadian Scholars Press Inc; 1989.
13. https://www.ons.org/practice-resources/competencies.
14. Ustjanauska AE, Bredice M, Nuhaily S, Kath L, Wells KJ. Training in patient navigation: a review of the research literature. Health Promot Pract. 2016;3:373–81.
15. Martinez, et al. Transforming the delivery of care in the post-healthcare reform era: what role will community health workers play? Am J Public Health. 2011;101:e1–5.
16. Whitley EM, Drisko J, Everhart RM, Samuels BA. Standardized academic education prepares competent community health workers. Am J Health Studies. 2007;22:121–6.
17. Rodolfo ER, Bent RJ, Eisman E, Nelsen PD, Rehm L and Richie P. A cube model for competency development: implications for psychology educators and regulators. Prof Psychol: Res Pract 2005;26:347–354.
18. Baldwin TT, Ford JK. Transfer of training: a review and directions for future research. Pers Psychol. 1988;41:63–105.
19. Freeman HP. The history, principles, and future of patient navigation: commentary. Seminol Oncol Nurs. (2013);29(2):72–5.
20. Accelerating Disparity Reducing Advances: Patient navigator program overview. Institute for alternative futures, 100 North Pitt Street, Alexandria, VA 22314, 2007.

Chapter 4
Steps to Successful Patient Navigation Programs

Angelina Esparza and Linda Fleisher

Starting at the Beginning: Steps to Successful Patient Navigation Programs

The old adage that if "you have seen one navigation program, you've seen one navigation program" speaks to the reality that each program needs to be designed based on the unique aspects of your organization, patient population and identified objectives for improving patient care. Creating and implementing a unique program based on best practices of the field and sound program planning principles will allow you to create an evidenced-based program tailored to your unique environment. Therefore, the time and effort spent before implementation in assessment and planning is well spent.

Program planning is crucial to allow time for clearly articulating your goals, understanding the costs associated with the program, preparing your organization to accept your ideas, developing your evaluation approach and measureable outcomes that have meaning both to your administration and patients and providing the foundation for successful implementation and evaluation.

There are five key steps to designing, implementing and evaluating your patient navigation program from Getting Started through Sustaining Your Program (Fig. 4.1).

The steps outlined are the ideal sequence, however, often it is difficult (if not impossible) to go through each step in a linear fashion. Many times, as a program

A. Esparza (✉)
Houston Health Department, 8000 North Stadium Drive, Houston, TX 77054, USA
e-mail: angelinae678@yahoo.com; Angelina.esparza@houstontx.gov

L. Fleisher
Department of Population Science, Fox Chase Cancer Center, 1318 Bradford Road, Oreland, PA 19075, USA
e-mail: fleisherl@email.chop.edu

E.A. Calhoun and A. Esparza (eds.), *Patient Navigation*,
DOI 10.1007/978-1-4939-6979-1_4

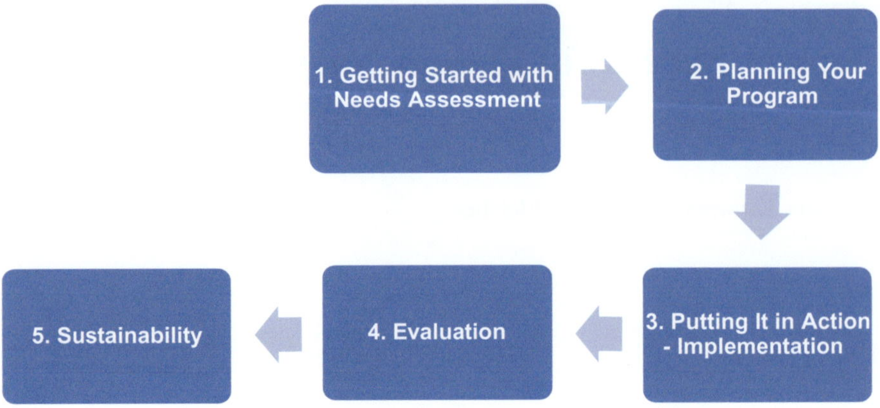

Fig. 4.1 Five key steps to successful planning, implementation and evaluation

planner, one must start somewhere in the middle of the process without the advantage of completing the previous steps, like completing a community and or needs assessment or understanding your organizational readiness. Often planning necessitates the need to re-evaluate and respond appropriately by modifying the original plan in response to new information, change in leadership and organizational focus, and as one assesses organizational readiness. It is never too late in the game to refine and enhance aspects of your program to achieve your goals. In the authors' experiences, if the program has stalled or has not been successful, one of these steps may have been omitted.

This chapter provides the roadmap to program planning and implementation and focuses on the foundations for implementation, such as organizational readiness and sustainability. These 5 steps can be addressed through a variety of simple to very complex approaches. Program planning and implementation is an iterative and evolving process and other chapters provide more depth and detail on critical areas such as needs assessment, models of navigation and evaluation.

Where to find more detail about specific steps in this book:

- Needs assessment to define your audience and the needs of your organization (see Chap. 2)
- Determining specific and measureable goals (see in this chapter)
- Defining your navigation model and approach (see Chap. 1)
- Choosing implementation strategies and identifying potential challenges, implementation and testing (Chap. 3)
- Designing and completing an evaluation and developing ongoing program monitoring and success measures (see in this chapter).

STEP 1—GETTING STARTED WITH YOUR ORGANIZATONAL NEEDS ASSESSMENT

1. Understanding Your Organization's Readiness

Assessing organizational readiness for program implementation is a key aspect to program planning and delivery. The assessment provides the opportunity to develop and share your vision and plan, understand the current infrastructure, capacity, and strengths of your organization, as well as identify and resolve potential challenges. The organizational assessment should not be confused with the program evaluation, but rather is part of the pre-implementation planning process. The assessment should address how to align the goals of the proposed program, in this case patient navigation, with the mission of the organization, existing workflows and programs, and potential support for the new service delivery model. Information should be gathered to consider the organizational structure and resource capacity (funding, training, space, patient flow, information technology, market trends, etc.) and determine the organizational psychology of readiness allowing for input from various organizational levels, from leadership to front line staff.

This stage allows for insights into whether or not the institution (hospital, clinic, etc.) is ready for the program. This assessment should be comprehensive and include an understanding of current practice, values and culture of the organization. Examine all aspects of the organization that might affect program development and implementation which might include the following: leadership understanding of the program and support, available resources (staffing, funding, reporting), organizational policies and politics, professional acceptance, and communication. This stage also provides the opportunity to identify barriers and assess the feasibility of the program. The end result is an environmental scan which will be the foundation for your program plan, implementation approach (including a timeline and process to facilitate the integration of your program into the system) and evaluation. Creating flexibility in your program plan will allow you to make small modifications while still achieving long-term goals of navigation and allow movement to the next phase, program installation.

Not only is this best practice, but recent research in the field of Implementation Science provides new insights into the understanding of organizational readiness and the value of addressing these organizational factors to increase successful implementation. Weiner (2009) described a theory of organizational readiness for change as a multi-faceted, multi-level construct, and includes both organizational commitment and efficacy (confidence) to change [1]. Two concepts are important ***structural readiness*** *(logistical and infrastructure needs)* and the ***psychological readiness*** (confidence and motivation) to implement change. Structural readiness is the best way to determine performance ability of the organization, current resources and capacity. Psychological assessment of readiness is necessary to understand staff feelings about their desire or need to change current practice and how successful they believe that change can be and if improvement is possible and necessary. Starting with structural readiness is often easier as it is concrete and can be easier to identify resources and needs.

Structural Readiness

This structural assessment will help to identify challenges and highlight the resources that are available to support implementation of patient navigation as well as provide an opportunity to clarify needs, develop communication tools, garner support, and become well informed about your institution.

Considerations in your structural assessment

- Space for staff
- Current staffing structure
- Role of patient navigator(s) in the patient flow process
- Role and responsibilities of the staff and how is it distinguished from others in the system.
- Funding to support the program
- Programmatic oversight and reporting structure
- Program communication and marketing
- Training and mentorship
- Resources for evaluation, reporting, and monitoring

Psychological Readiness

Once the structural readiness is determined it is equally important to determine the psychological readiness of the organization to adopt and adjust to the proposed change. Three main concepts are key to understanding change at this level:

- change efficacy
- change motivation
- change commitment

While structural assessment details the capacity for change, psychological assessment help to determine the confidence that the organization (efficacy) can implement the program successfully and determine the level if understanding as to why the change is needed and the benefit(s) of change (motivation). Assessing psychological readiness is a multi-layered and dependent on various levels of engagement and a shared understanding and mutually agreed upon outcomes and a shared vision for improvement.

Change efficacy increases when there is a collective sense of confidence in the organization that the change can occur successfully, that the collective team has some level of selectiveness in the process. When organizational efficacy is high, organizational members (staff) are more likely to initiate and adopt change and program implementation, exert greater effort to support the change, exhibit increased persistence in the face of challenges, and display the cooperative behavior. These factors can help to foster and result in effective implementation. [1, 2] The group perceives that the implementation will bring about positive change and it can be successful. Weiner (2009) proposes that determining organizational efficacy is dependent on three factors: tasks demands, resource availability, and situational factors [1].

Considerations in your psychological assessment

- Does the organization know what it will take to implement change and program effectively?
- Are the resources to implement the program available?
- Can the organization implement given the current organizational environment? (competition, staffing, patient load, other environmental change, past experience with change)
- Is this a bottom up or top down initiative?
- Is there ways to create consensus?
- Are there regulatory or marketing drivers?

Organizational motivation should be assessed, particularly at the individual level and lower levels across the organization. Motivation can be summarized by the following:

- If a decision has been determined by leadership and staff feel they have little or no choice to adopt the resulting changes. The staff will often feel that they "must or have to change".
- The staff may see the need for a change and have input into the change and feel that elicited feedback is part of the plan. This creates a feeling of personal input and is often characterized by supporting a feeling of "wanting to change".
- External factors push the organization to change or practice change happens at the professional level and staff may feel they "ought to change".

The most beneficial motivation to support program implementation is the commitment or "want to change". This implies that the staff and organization has weighed the needs and benefits and supports the change to current structure to improve the outcomes outlined. In other words, the "value" of the program is viewed as beneficial and the motivation to implement change is high. Achieving this level of buy in will most likely take some work to accomplish successfully and in reality there may be a mix of all three motivations which ultimately brings about change. Inevitably, different part of the organization may also vary in their motivation, but if the majority and the change/program champion are ready create a fertile environment for implementation.

So, the best way to assure organizational efficacy, motivation and commitment is to develop a clear plan based on input from all levels so it reflects the organizational readiness and engenders support by key organizational stakeholders. Make sure the plan addresses the values and necessary outcomes to move the collective towards the actions necessary for change. This can be done by developing a strong business case for support, conducting staff and stakeholder briefings.

You can complete your plan after this assessment or modify your current plan to address the challenges and strengths discovered in organizational assessment, ultimately building the confidence for successful implementation. Using past experiences of successful change in the organization can bolster your position.

Therefore, the need for a comprehensive structural assessment, understanding the capacity, and the perception (psychological) of the staff is important to bridge the perception and reality of implementation. The task is to assure that the staff is confident about the human, financial, material and informational resources, time and political environment necessary for successful implementation [1].

2. Conducting an organizational assessment for patient navigation

There are three phases of organizational assessment: (1) information gathering, (2) gathering input, (3) develop a statement of need [3].

(1) *Information gathering* can include information about where and how patient navigation might be most successfully integrated in your organization and often integrates gathering input as well. The information in these two first steps then can help to complete the third and fourth steps to create a more refined and tailored program plan to benefit your institution. One should try and research all aspects of the organization and how navigation may be useful in improving outcomes and support staff in achieving their short and long—term goals.

Through information gathering one can discuss the concept with others to evaluate the comprehension of patient navigation, how the group envisions and defines navigation, and what benefits might be derived from developing a program. Equally as important, and often where there is more to learn, is what might be some anticipated challenges, misbeliefs, or concerns related to navigation. This allows the program planner to proceed and start to understand what data, education, or discussion might be necessary to create a fertile environment for an open discussion. Additionally, the information gathering can help one identify internal champions to support the implantation and are willing to work with the planner. These champions, as discussed later, can help to bolster support at all levels. The information gathering should be a both formal (gathering input) and informal (lunch time discussions and co-workers conversations). All of the information gathered in this phase will help to determine the best data to gather in a more formal process (surveys, interviews, review of patient data, etc.) Additionally, this phase will help you determine the initial structural and psychological readiness for implementation.

Methods to collect data include, but are not limited to the following

(1) Key Informant Interviews (staff, patients, administrators, etc.)
(2) Surveys (written or questionnaire)
(3) Focus groups
(4) Review of patient and systems data (to identify specific need and are for improvement)
(5) Community data and needs assessment
(6) Literature review and identification of best practices
(7) Information from professional organizations and other non-profits who might be able to offer guidance and advice

(2) *Gathering input* should include various levels of the organization from patients to leadership and should not only include individual level data but should include groups, units, departments, etc. This can be done either formally (focus groups and surveys) or informally (general feedback, informal discussions, etc.) Consider these questions: What do the patients we serve need and how can patient navigation address this need? How, specifically, will the implementation of your proposed program answer this need? What is the goal and mission of the institution and how does your program plan align with those of the institution? What are staff perceptions of the role of the patient navigator? Is the patient navigator viewed as a threat or a needed resource? Is leadership ready to embrace the needed changes and publically support the program?

(3) *Statement of need* Once information is gathered, then what? It is important to clearly articulate the statement of need or problem statement which the program will address since the statement will become a focal point for the type of navigation program to be implemented. There is information available through the Centers for Disease Control and Prevention that provide helpful guidance on creating a problem statement. http://www.cdc.gov/healthcommunication/cdcynergy/problemdescription.html.

Recall the information gathering and think about the reason you, the planner believes that patient navigation will solve a problem or enhance outcomes. After speaking with your colleagues and gathering information did you find the need to re-evaluate your first premise? Once you gather the information you should be able to develop a statement of need. This is a sentence or two that summarizes the why the community, patients, system, etc. would benefit from patient navigation and how (briefly) the benefit will be derived. So with this in mind, as data and information is being gathered think about what you need to create and or support your statement of need and how navigation would provide the stated benefit/improvement.

Example: Statement of Need

Survivorship Care Plans have been challenging to implement with existing workflows and limited staffing and are critical for ongoing care for patients. Therefore, a survivorship patient navigation program is being implemented to fill this gap.

3. Community Assessment—Understanding client needs

Just as we have explored the needs and structure of our organization to carefully design our navigation program, it is critical to decide what specific audience will be served (e.g. specific cancer site, stage of disease, survivorship) and then more fully understand the audience's specific needs. Before you begin to develop your navigation program, you need to clearly articulate who you are serving and at what point of care. You also need to fully understand the needs of your community and patients in order to design a program that is responsive and ultimately successful. Although you may have experience with your communities and patients and believe you know their needs, it is essential that you reach out to them directly and ask.

Chapter 1 provides valuable information on the purpose of a needs assessment and the various approaches. Knowing who your audience is allows you to determine the scope of your needs assessment, whether it is a community wide assessment, an assessment of your patients or both. The model presented by Dr. Suarez-Balcazar highlights the steps in the Community Needs Assessment Process and is linked the overall program plan. Your program plan is what allows you to act on the needs assessment data.

As part of the needs assessment process there are other data sources that you might use to help you more fully understand the needs of your patients. If you are hospital based, your patient satisfaction surveys may provide insight to areas of improvement. Or find out who in your organization is responsible for your IRS mandated Community Benefit Community Needs Assessment or your required Cancer Committee Needs Assessment. Typically there are other departments or groups in your organization who may have data or conducting similar assessments that could be an important resource. Often, we don't need to recreate the wheel, but review these reports and data in light of our goal in designing and implementing a patient navigation program. For programs to make an impact, they need to include the perspective of the consumer.

Considerations for Community Needs Assessments

- Is the program focusing on women in the community who have not been participating in cancer screening and our goal is to navigate them into screening services?
- Is the gap in the health care organization at the point of treatment and the time between a call for an appointment and the first visit?
- Or is the program focusing on diabetic care and the need is to navigate patients through various providers and health care organizations?
- Or is the program focusing on comprehensive navigation from screening to survivorship?
- Will the program focus only on the underserved or for all clients?

If there is a large Immigrant population, how will we handle translation services?

4. Identifying and troubleshooting challenges—Adaptation of the plan based on feedback

The information gathered in the steps listed above should be used to determine areas in which the organization may readily adopt the innovation, i.e. the need for the patient navigator. One must determine if the concept is well understood, supported by staff and leadership and if there exists areas that need further consideration, i.e. funding, staffing and training. Completing the original needs assessment has determined the scope of work of the patient navigator within your system (Chap. 2). In the community assessment, you should have determined the desired outcome of you program as well as a proposed response based on the population needs. With those pieces firmly in place, we can now explore how to align the needs of your community with the organization and determine a mismatch or gaps.

There are some common challenges that many navigation programs have experienced including role delineation, mismatch between the organization's and patients' goals and expectations, organizational structure (who will manage the program), budgeting, data management concerns (including linking to existing systems) and plans for sustainability. The needs assessment process should uncover these issues and allow time to successfully problem solve these issues. For example, there may be conflict about where the navigation program should align e.g. nursing, social work, community outreach) and there is not necessary a right or wrong answer. However, reviewing the agreed upon objectives and goals may help to make this a decision based on need not preference. Talking with other navigators or navigator administrators from other organizations can also provide insights into how these conflicts were handled and resolved. There is a growing number of patient navigation professional groups and organizations that can be important resources.

5. Improving the system and outcomes

At this point one should have sufficient problem statement, be able to clearly articulate how navigation will solve the problem or improve the system and what challenges and champions you have within your environment. The next suggested step understanding how clients access and utilize your system and where in that process navigation may be able to help. This is an important consideration and often given little thought prior to implementation.

Many hospitals may refer to this process as patient/client flow. In some cases the organization may have painstaking detail on how a patient enters the system and accesses needed services. In other cases, the process may not be as clear. As the planner, one must review the current process, identify where the navigator will be introduced and how they will be integrated into the existing process or modify the process as needed. Failure to dedicate careful consideration of the process can result in improper introduction of navigation services, perhaps too late in the process to be most useful to the clients or too early, before patients have time to understand their diagnosis and perhaps anticipate needs.

The placement of the navigator should be tied to the intended outcomes of the program, the number of navigators, budget and training of the navigator. Additionally, practical issues such as supervision and budget or acceptance of the program may dictate the entry point into the process system. Be aware that often placement isn't ideal for political reasons and may be modified later as data can be gathered that would identify the best point for integration.

Step 2: PLANNING YOUR PROGRAM—Starting at the beginning while keeping your eye on the end goal.

Planning is essential to long term success and it is critical to include your evaluation approach as part of the initial planning process. There are many planning models that can guide the development, implementation and evaluation of your patient navigation program. These include simple to very complex approaches, but no matter the complexity a number of key components are important.

Now that you have completed your organizational and community needs assessment, it is time to develop a program plan which includes:

- specific and measureable goals
- your navigation model and approach
- implementation strategies and potential challenges
- evaluation approach

Although these steps seem easy to address, we often make assumptions about those we are trying to serve and underestimate the challenges to implementation.

According to the Institute of Medicine, "a well-thought out plan extends throughout the lifespan of your project…and helps guide the development process by providing objectives, by setting priorities, and mapping out tasks." [4] There are many planning models and tools that you can use to guide the development, implementation and evaluation of your patient navigation program [4–12].

There are a number of things to consider in your planning process, including:

- What are the goals and objectives of the program? Do you have short and long term goals?
- What type of model of navigation will be used and how does this link back to the organizational and community assessment?
- Where will the program fit within the organization?
- What is the role of the navigator in your program? What orientation & training will be required?
- What type of evaluation will you conduct? What types of data collection is needed? How will you monitor and track the program?

1. Goals and Objectives

The goal(s) of program are typically a broad, general statement about the problem you are trying to address. Whereas your objectives are measurable and specific actions that define what you plan on achieving. There can be different types of objectives such as those that address activities (process objectives), or short or long term changes in behavior or outcomes (impact and outcome objectives). Since objectives are measurable, they should be linked to your evaluation so you know if you have met your objective.

Clear objectives are the key for program planning and evaluation and not always articulated in our planning process. One strategy for developing well-written objectives is the use the SMART approach. *For example, in 2013, we will navigate a minimum of 200 women with abnormal mammograms into their first follow-up appointment within 10 days of their abnormal result letter being sent.* Additional objectives could articulate other components of the program, such as *100% of women who are navigated and need translation services will be provided qualified interpreters at their first follow-up appointment.* SMART objectives require us to think through what specifically we are trying to accomplish and what needs to be measured. It also allows us to ensure that our objectives are addressing the overall goal of the program. In this case above, the overall goal is to reduce the number of women who do not have timely follow-up to an abnormal mammogram.

SMART Objectives

Specific
Measurable
Attainable/Achievable
Relevant
Time bound

2. Role of the Navigator

In addition to deciding the role of the navigator and type of model (clinical, community), it is important to develop a very specific job description both to communicate internally and support the navigator in defining their responsibilities. The job description will also be an important tool in the hiring process. During the interviewing process it is important to have your internal stakeholders participate in the interviews and provide feedback on the candidates. Developing a set of behavioral questions regarding real world situations and how their experience fits these situations especially focused on communication and managing conflict, will provide insights into how the candidate might handle this very challenging role. One lesson from our own experience is the make sure the candidate can handle a hospital based setting. Although someone may have the personality and skill to be an exceptional community navigator, they may be uncomfortable in a hospital setting with very sick patients.

And, even with the most qualified candidate, the orientation and training process is critical to success. A carefully designed orientation, with input from the various departments and groups within the organization that will be involved with the navigation program, will ensure the new navigator understands the organizational structure, identify resources and support, and assimilate into their "connector" role. Many orientation and training manuals, articles and programs are available and Chap. 1 discusses this issue in more detail.

3. Planning Models and Tools

There are many planning models out there in public health, nursing and health care related fields. Some of the key elements we have already addressed, such as conducting a needs assessment, understanding the organizational environment and developing program goals and objectives.

A tool that is often used in program planning is called a Logic Model or a Theory Model. It is a way to diagram your program and its intended impact and outcomes. Logic Models are a way of linking program goals, objectives, activities and outcomes. They are a map that can easily communicate the program. They show the if-then process, if we do this activity, we expect this result. These logic models can be rather simple or very complex, and there are many resources available to develop logic models. The key to a logic model is to start from the end. What is your outcome? What do you expect your program to accomplish? Then, what are the short term changes that need to happen both at the patient, provider and system level to accomplish this outcome? What behavior or knowledge change to we expect? What are the barriers and facilitators that our program will address?

In regards to evaluation, many times we don't plan the evaluation until the program is well underway. But, although the actual process of evaluation occurs during and after implementation, the planning of the evaluation ideally should occur at this planning stage. The evaluation should provide the evidence to show that the program is meeting the objectives and provide insights into how to improve the program. It should also provide the information that you and your organization requires for sustainability. Evaluations do not need to be complex if your resources are limited. A simple plan that highlights each metric for each objective and then a process to collect the data for that metric is a good starting place. Some programs have used simple excel sheets to keep these data, while others have built or bought data management systems. It is also helpful to align the evaluation with other evaluation efforts, such as patient satisfaction or community benefit. Creating those linkages will help you to leverage limited resources. Some questions to consider in your planning process include:

- What data can be collected to determine if we are meeting our goals? How many patients were approached and received navigation services in a timely fashion?
- What data can be collected to understand what services are being delivered? What kinds of issues are navigators addressing? How much time does it take? How many encounters? What types of referrals?
- Who will collect the data? What is the impact on the navigator's time?
- What data are available that can be used? Does the medical record include dates to determine time from diagnosis to start of treatment?
- Do we have the resources for a comprehensive data management system? What are the resources within the institution?
- How often do we need to report and to whom?

A good rule of thumb is to only collect the data you are going to use in supporting and improving your program.

Program Planning Resources

Public Health
Precede-Proceed
NACCHO, Mobilizing for Action through Planning and Partnerships (MAPP)
http://www.naccho.org/topics/infrastructure/MAPP/index.cfm
Healthy People 2020
http://healthypeople.gov/2020/
Cancer Control Plans
http://cancercontrolplanet.cancer.gov/state_plans.jsp
Community Tool Box
http://ctb.ku.edu/en/tablecontents/index.aspx
Nursing and Health Care
HEDIS Measures http://www.ncqa.org/HEDISQualityMeasurement/HEDISMeasures.aspx
Logic Models—Center for Disease Control and Prevention
http://www.cdc.gov/oralhealth/state_programs/pdf/logic_models.pdf
Minnesota Department of Health
http://www.health.state.mn.us/divs/opi/qi/toolbox/logic.html
Community Toolbox

http://ctb.ku.edu/en/table-of-contents/overview/models-for-community-health-and-development/logic-model-development/main

Step 3: PUTTING IT IN ACTION [13]

Implementing any program in a system should be planned with sufficient detail to clearly articulate the goals and objectives of the program, scope of the navigation practice, and the desired outcome of the intervention. The outcomes of the intervention are important, but of equal importance should be an implementation strategy to assure success. Often the term evidence based practice is used, however, evidence based implementation should be an important consideration.

There are some approaches to consider:

- Gradients of implementation including pilot testing, phase in process and full integration
- Marketing and promotion—internal and external
- Clear management plan and roles/responsibilities
- Staffing assessments and continuing education and professional development
- Reporting and record keeping
- Keeping stakeholders engaged
- Quality Improvement Plans—patient and provider satisfaction, problem solving

Many programs have found it helpful to start small. For example, starting with a pilot program in one clinic area or a specific point in the patient flow (e.g. entry into the system or post-treatment) and then phase in the program in other areas before having a comprehensive program can provide important insights about management, record-keeping, training, building support and promotion. These early learnings and success can build the momentum and show the return on investment early on.

The implementation approach should address organizational factors (reporting and supervision, budget, staffing structure, data management, space), navigator role (responsibilities, reporting, initial and ongoing training, professional development) and patient expectations and feedback (patient satisfaction As patient navigation is a relatively new field of healthcare providers need to clearly understand the scope and intent of the patient navigator and understand how it will fit into the current patient flow and case finding. Often established systems within hospitals may oppose a new change to the patient flow.

Step 4: EVALUATION

Understanding if your program worked as intended and whether or not you reached your objectives is the primary focus of evaluation and is critical whether it is to report back to your organizational leadership to maintain support of your navigation program and services, make improvements in your program (Quality Improvement Goals), determine how best to expand your program or even publish your results in professional or scientific journals. It is essential that evaluation be built in at the program planning phase and be tied directly to your program objectives. We know that some of the evaluation data will be to meet reporting requirements for your organization, but there are many other valuable opportunities to utilize these data. And important point, is to only collect data that you will use being in your evaluation. It is a burden to patients and staff to collect and maintain programmatic data, so choose wisely and share your findings back with your stakeholders as well. It will help them see the value of this information. Also determine any organizational policies or requirements for data collection, such as HIPPA or Human Subjects Protection (IRB). And finally, explore various approaches to collecting and storing the data, either through existing data management systems within your institution or developing your own systems (including Excel files depending on your resources and IT support).

There are multiple levels of evaluation that correspond to your levels of objectives, namely: process, impact and outcome.

- Process evaluation focuses on answering questions about the implementation of the program. Was it implemented as intended? Were the barriers to implementation? Were patients and providers satisfied with the program or services? What was the cost of navigation?
- Impact evaluation focuses on short-term effects of the program. For example, did the program improve time to diagnosis, proportion of women screened, retention rates, knowledge of patients and providers? What is the downstream revenue capture?
- Outcome evaluation focuses on longer term impacts, such as reduction in late stage disease, reductions in morbidity or mortality.

For many navigator programs, process and impact evaluation are most feasible and appropriate to guide the implementation and quality improvement strategies. For many programs, sustainability is a challenge and the economic data measuring the cost of the program and the potential downstream revenue is critical. Many programs have shown that there is a decrease in lost to follow-up or an increase in patient caseloads which impact downstream revenue. These data can be very important to show that the program is cost neutral or even revenue producing.

Step 5: SUSTAINABILITY

Maintaining support can be a difficult task given the many competing patient support needs and potential initiatives to improve health outcomes and the patient experience. While you have implemented your program successfully, it is no time to stop planning. Now as a successful program director, it is your responsibility to assure continued support (financial and other) to maintain and improve/expand the program. You must continuously create the business case for continuing the program. You should be able to accomplish building the business case because you have taken the previous steps of defining the problem, tailoring your approach to fit and support the functions of your organization, identified best practices to implement and data collection. In addition, because you have tested your strategies first, and then grown the program, you have the information you need to effectively communicate the value of patient navigation in your system.

Programs are most effective, often, when they can be sustained overtime. Allocation of resources is often a barrier to continued implementation. In order to assure that resources and support are continuously provided, one must recognize the crucial elements in program sustainability. It is also important to recognize that taking steps in your daily work to incorporate activities to build sustainability.

Schell et al. [14] conducted a study reviewing sustainability models to identify the core components. Their work included a literature review, input from and expert panel and concept mapping process to identify the core domains of sustainability in public health programs. The end result is a framework which clearly articulates the key elements to keep in mind to develop a business case and resource justification within your organization.

Sustainability discussions should include a number of key aspects. While often the discussion is around finances, other factors should be included, such as:

(1) Outcomes and Evaluation- Did you measure the right, best and most feasible outcomes
(2) Support- How supportive was the environment and was the organizational readiness challenges addressed or does more work need to be accomplished to increase political and organizational support?
(3) Partnerships- Where the right partners (internal and external) at the table and was the interaction between and across system successful?
(4) Communications- How were success of the program communicated to the various end-users and stakeholders? What needs to be improved?
(5) Planning and future growth – How will the program change or grow? Are there anticipated changes that need to be taken into account moving forward?

Summary

As the program developer you should communicate effectively the statement of need (community, system, population, etc.) and how the program has improved the challenge or added value to the system, patient experience, etc. In addition to communicating for the purpose of obtaining resources, communication should be used to effectively inform about the activities and accomplishments of the patient navigator program. One should also work continuously on quality improvement of the program, which is accomplished through effective implementation and evaluation and adapted as needed. Collaboration and partnerships should be ongoing and allows for networking, sharing of resources and support (political and otherwise). Using a structured framework as you begin to conceptualize your program and implement will help not only guide your work to success it will also provide the justification and evidence you need to convey the importance of sustaining your program over time.

With this step by step roadmap to designing and evaluating you are ready. Use the checklist to help you keep track of the process and the subsequent chapters for more detailed discussion and guidance.

Key Steps Checklist

Step 1—Getting Started With Your Needs Assessment

- Have you conducted talked with stakeholders in your organization? Do you understand the challenges you may face? Have you identified champions at all levels?
- How has your organization addressed other innovations or new programs?
- How would you rate your organizational readiness for a patient navigation program
- Have you identified the need for the program? What data do you have to support the need for the program?
- Have you reviewed other needs assessment reports or materials from your organization, e.g. the required Community Needs Assessment for Hospitals?
- Have you reviewed the current clinical or patient workflow to determine how your program can easily be integrated?
- Have you identified key organizational barriers & facilitators to acceptance, start-up and implementation?
- Have you started to think about what might be important for evaluation and sustainability?

Step 2—Planning Your Program

- Have you developed your program goals and SMART objectives? Have you shared them with key stakeholders and addressed their feedback?
- Have you carefully considered the various models of navigation, e.g. clinical vs non-clinical?
- What are the key performance standards that navigators will be measured for success? What type of background is required for these KPI's? What is the required background for navigators (e.g. nurse, social work, community outreach)? Are there linguistic or cultural background requirements?
- What will your training and orientation program look like?
- Should you start as a pilot or full implementation?
- Where does the program fit organizationally? Who will manage the program?
- What resources and budget are required?

Step 3—Putting it into Action

- Have you planned a launch of your program, including key stakeholders?
- Do you have an advisory and schedule of meetings?
- Do you have promotional or marketing materials?

- Are there other programs or departments that need to be oriented to the program since it may impact their work flow, requires coordination or would be making referrals?
- What kind of supervisory process is in place? Are targets and goals being met? Are the needs of the navigators being met?

Step 4—Evaluation

- Do you have an evaluation plan—addressing implementation, patient satisfaction, staff satisfaction, and outcomes?
- How will you track the navigation program—e.g. case load, quality assurance?
- How will you track impact and outcomes? Use an existing database? Build a database? Integrate into patient satisfaction surveys?
- How, if at all, will your data collection be linked or integrated into the current IT systems (e.g. EMR)
- What kinds of reports (operating and outcome) will you need? To whom and how often
- Do you plan on publishing your results? Are there any human subjects' requirements?

Step 5—Sustainability

- What is the budget cycle in your institution to ensure the program is part of the process?
- What are the key KPI's that your institution needs to continue supporting the program?
- Are there external grants or funding opportunities to explore?
- Should the program be expanded? Why or why not?
- What kinds of continuing education efforts are in place? Conferences, journal clubs?
- Are there innovations in patient navigation field to consider (e.g. use of technology, certification standards, expansion into other conditions)
- Is the program being promoted? Do staff and patients know it exists? Do you need to refine or expand your promotional efforts?

References

1. Weiner B. A theory of organizational readiness for change. Implement. Sci. [Internet]. 2009 October [cited 10 Feb 2016]; 4(1). Available from http://vv4kg5gr5v.search.serialssolutions.com.libproxy.temple.edu/?sid=Entrez:PubMed&id=pmid:19840381.
2. Shea C, Jacobs S, Esserman D, Bruce K, Weiner B. Organizational readiness for implementing change: a psychometric assessment of a new measure. Implement. Sci. 2014; [cited 16 Feb 2016]; 9(7).
3. Cancer Patient Navigation Program Toolkit [Internet]. Kansas Cancer Partnership; 2009 [cited 16 Feb 2016]. Available from http://www.cancerkansas.org/toolkit.htm.

4. Smart Bites Toolkit [Internet]. Institutes of Medicine; [cited 16 Feb 2016]. Available from http://www.google.com/url?sa=t%26rct=j%26q=%26esrc=s%26source=web%26cd=1%26ved=0ahUKEwjV_NThz-jKAhWICpAKHSO9BUQQFggcMAA%26url=http%3A%2F%2Fiom.nationalacademies.org%2FAbout-IOM%2FMaking-a-Difference%2FCommunity-Outreach%2F ~ %2Fmedia%2FFiles%2FAbout%2520the%2520IOM%2FSmartBites%2FSmartBitesToolkit.pdf%26usg=AFQjCNEggxSfe2Eo8d-3pZdt9gDCRxTj0g%26bvm=bv.113370389,d.cWw.
5. National Association of County & City Health Officials. Mobilizing for action through planning and partnerships [Internet]. Washington, DC: National Association of County and City Health Officials; 2016 [cited 16 Feb 2016]. Available from http://www.naccho.org/topics/infrastructure/MAPP/index.cfm.
6. Healthy People 2020 [Internet]. Washington, DC: U.S. Department of Health and Human Services, Office of Disease Prevention and Health Promotion; 2016 [cited 16 Feb 2016]. Available from http://healthypeople.gov/2020/.
7. Cancer Control P.L.A.N.E.T. State, Tribe, and Territory Plans. [Internet]. Division of Cancer Control and Population Sciences at National Cancer Institute; 2016 [cited 16 Feb 2016]. Available from http://cancercontrolplanet.cancer.gov/state_plans.jsp.
8. NCQA. HEDIS Measures [Internet]. NCQA; 2016 [cited 16 Feb 2016]. Available from http://www.ncqa.org/HEDISQualityMeasurement/HEDISMeasures.aspx.
9. Community Tool Box. Table of contents [Internet]. Kansas: Work Group for Community Health and Development; 2015 [cited 16 Feb 2016]. Available from http://ctb.ku.edu/en/tablecontents/index.aspx.
10. Community Tool Box-Developing a Logic Model or Theory of change [Internet]. Kansas: Work Group for Community Health and Development; 2015 [cited 16 Feb 2016]. Available from http://ctb.ku.edu/en/table-of-contents/overview/models-for-community-health-and-development/logic-model-development/main.
11. Logic Models [Internet]. Centers for disease control and prevention; [cited 16 Feb 2016]. Available from http://www.cdc.gov/oralhealth/state_programs/pdf/logic_models.pdf.
12. Logic Model—QI Toolbox—Minnesota Dept. of Health [Internet]. [Cited 16 Feb 2016]. Available from: http://www.health.state.mn.us/divs/opi/qi/toolbox/logic.html.
13. Parkinson & Associates. Managing health promotion in the workforce: guidelines for implementation and evaluation. Palo Alto, CA: Mayfield; 1982.
14. Schell SF, Luke DA, Schooley MW, Elliott MB, Herbers SH, Mueller NB, Bunger AC. Public health program capacity for sustainability: a new framework. Implement Sci. 2013;1(8):15. doi:10.1186/1748-5908-8-15.

Chapter 5
Program Evaluation

Elizabeth A. Calhoun and Betsy C. Risendal

Introduction

Program evaluation is an essential organizational practice in public health; however, it is not practiced consistently across program areas, nor is it sufficiently well integrated into the day-to-day management of most programs. Program evaluation is also necessary for guiding public health activities, which include (a) using science as a basis for decision-making and public health action; (b) expanding the quest for social equity through public health action; (c) performing effectively as a service agency; (d) making efforts outcome oriented; and (e) being accountable. These operating principles imply several ways to improve how public health activities are planned and managed. They underscore the need for programs to develop clear plans, inclusive partnerships, and feedback systems that allow learning and ongoing improvement to occur. One way to ensure that new and existing patient navigation programs honor these principles is for each program to conduct routine, practical evaluations that provide information for management and improve program effectiveness.

What is Program Evaluation?

Program evaluations are individual, systematic studies that use objective measurement and analysis to answer specific questions about how well a program is working. Program evaluations also help to weigh the benefits of the program and

E.A. Calhoun (✉)
University of Arizona Health Sciences, 1350 N. Warren Avenue,
P.O. Box 245018, Tucson, AZ 85724, USA
e-mail: ecalhoun@email.arizona.edu

B.C. Risendal
Department of Community and Behavioral Health, Colorado School
of Public Health, 13001 E. 17th Place, Aurora, CO 80045, USA
e-mail: betsy.risendal@ucdenver.edu

E.A. Calhoun and A. Esparza (eds.), *Patient Navigation*,
DOI 10.1007/978-1-4939-6979-1_5

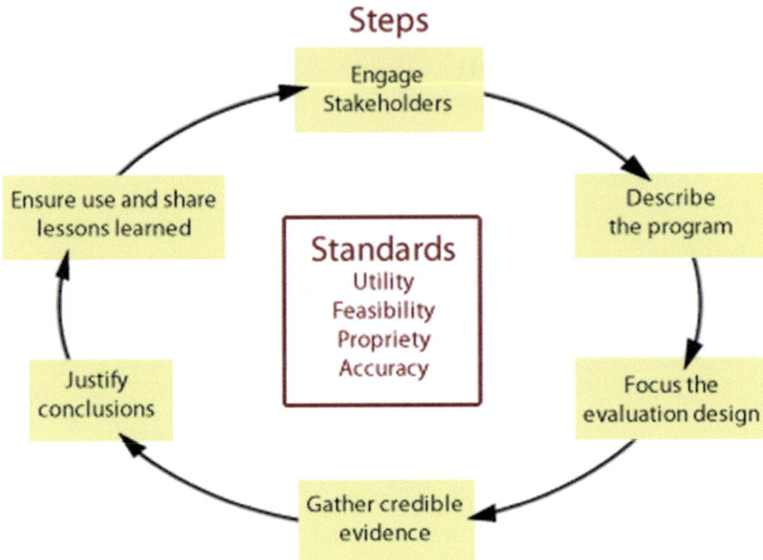
Steps
Engage Stakeholders
Describe the program
Focus the evaluation design
Gather credible evidence
Justify conclusions
Ensure use and share lessons learned
Standards
Utility
Feasibility
Propriety
Accuracy

Fig. 5.1 Schematic describing the steps involved in program evaluation

implement policy against its unintended outcomes and costs. Figure 5.1 illustrates the different steps involved in program evaluation.

Why Conduct Program Evaluation?

Many times program evaluation activities are conducted only because funders or institutions require it. Evaluation is often viewed as a distraction from the main purpose of the program. However, when program evaluation is planned and implemented carefully, the results can be very useful to maximize program potential as follows [1]:

- Who are the clients, and what are their needs?
- How can we demonstrate the impact and benefits of our program activities for sustainability?
- How do our activities compare to best practices in patient navigation, and how might we improve?

Benefits of Program Evaluation

- Supports continuous quality program improvement
- Increases understanding of the program—how are activities and strategies linked to results?
- Leads to improved planning and management
- Provides a better understanding of programs and what works

Defining a Program Evaluation

- A Program Plan is a road map for your activities
- The Plan must be based upon a plausible theory
- It facilitates your program's systematic implementation
- Ensure specific plans are made for each activity

Planning a Program

- Plan—What is the plan for this program?
- Process Evaluation—Does the program has high implementation fidelity?
- Outcome Evaluation—How well is the program working?
- CQI—What are the Continuous Quality Improvement strategies?
- Sustain—If the program was successful, how will it be sustained?

How Do I Decide What to Measure?

Each funded program is required to collect several pieces of information about the type of activities, the number of persons served by the program, and characteristics of persons served by the program. Below we will show how these data can be used to answer the questions posed above.

RE-AIM is a common evaluation framework (RE-AIM.org) that may be useful in guiding what to measure in patient navigation program evaluation [1]. The purpose of using this framework as a guide for what to collect is because it will help ensure that the program evaluation will be useful. Each letter in the acronym stands for the following:

- Reach: number, proportion, and representativeness of participants (and who is being missed)
- Effectiveness: results of program—does it make a short-term (impact) and/or long-term (outcome) difference
- Adoption: number, proportion, and representativeness of settings
- Implementation: fidelity to protocol/program goals, and use of best practices/strategies
- Maintenance: institutionalization (prove worth and benefit to organization), cost of implementation, and long-term effects.

What is Involved in Program Planning?

- Needs/Resources Assessment—what needs to be addressed?
- Set Goals—What are goals, target population, and objectives (i.e., desired outcomes)
- Best Practice—Decide on what evidence-based model is most useful in reaching goals
- Fit—What do you need to do to ensure your program 'fits' the community context
- Capacities—Organization capacities

What is a Needs Assessment?

- What problem is the program attempting to address?
- Whom does this program serve; to what extent are their needs met?
- What should be the documented goals of the program?

Developing a Logic Model

- A logic model, as demonstrated in Fig. 5.2 [2], establishes a relationship between problems being addressed, the activities employed to address them, and the expected outcomes
- A logic model creates program clarity, fosters a consensus among everyone involved, and helps identify inaccuracies in plan.

Designing a Program Evaluation

- What do you want to know? (key questions)
- Who will be involved in or affected by the evaluation or use the findings? (stakeholders)
- To focus an evaluation, consider its purpose, uses, questions, methods, roles, budgets, deliverables, etc.
- An evaluation cannot answer all questions for all stakeholders.

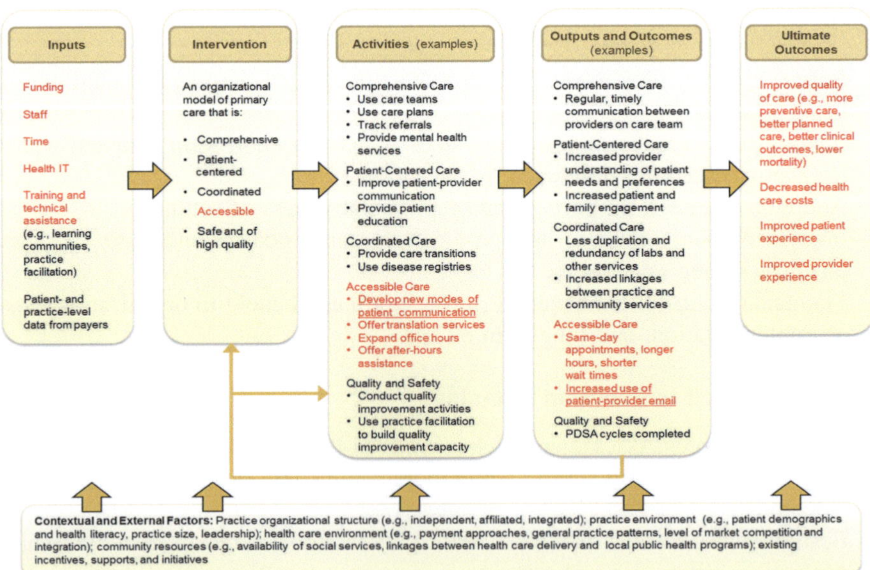

Fig. 5.2 Overarching medical home—logic model example. *Source* [2], U.S. Department of health and human services

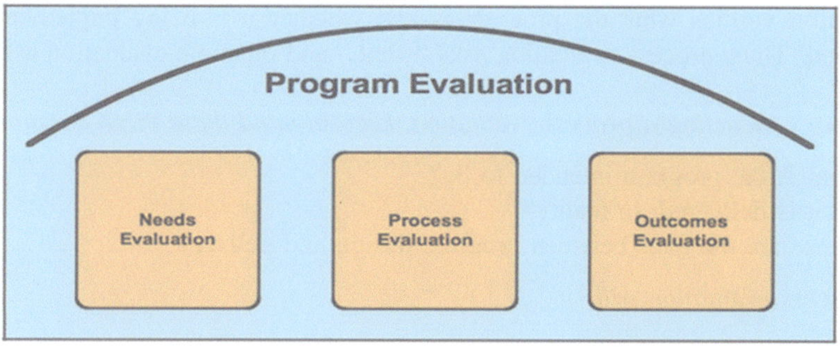

Fig. 5.3 Types of program evaluation

Types of Program Evaluation There are three main types of program evaluation, as illustrated in Fig. 5.3—Needs Evaluation, Process Evaluation, and Outcomes Evaluation. Each type of program evaluation is discussed in detail below.

Needs Evaluation Needs Assessment is a type of evaluation that is conducted before a program is designed (or re-designed). A Needs Assessment evaluation is conducted to gather information to determine if the proposed service is actually necessary, and how the service should be designed. There is no one standard list of questions that is considered in doing a Needs Assessment evaluation, but the following questions are typically considered. The issues and questions considered in Needs Assessment evaluation do not address what happens during a program, nor does the evaluation attempt to measure outcomes. Little statistical analysis is required for a Needs Assessment evaluation.

Types of Questions When Planning a Needs Evaluation:

- Is there a need for this kind of program? Are there other programs that are the same or similar?
- What are the characteristics of the clientele for whom the program is being designed (e.g., demographic characteristics, problem severity)?
- What is the estimated size of the "target" population?
- What is the estimated demand for and capacity of the program being designed?
- Are there particular barriers that the "target" population is likely to encounter in participating in the program?
- What are the staff and facilities that are required?
- Is there a "best practice" literature in this area?

Process Evaluation *What is process evaluation?*

Process evaluation uses empirical data to assess the delivery of programs. In contrast to outcome evaluation, which assesses the impact of the program, process evaluation verifies what the program is and whether it is being implemented as designed. Thus, process evaluation asks "what," and outcome evaluation asks, "so what?"

When conducting a process evaluation, keep in mind these three questions:

1. What is the program intended to be?
2. What is delivered, in reality?
3. Where are the gaps between program design and delivery?

Process evaluation will:

- Measure program fidelity
- Help you assess which activities were implemented
- Provide the strengths and weaknesses of implementation
- Allow you to make necessary changes/improvements
- Improve the overall program evaluation outcomes

Outcome Evaluation

An outcome evaluation investigates whether changes occur for participants in a program and if these changes are associated with a program or an activity. Such evaluations examine whether, to what extent, and in what direction outcomes change for those in the program. Outcomes are specific attitudes, knowledge, behaviors, or skills that programs aim to influence positively. Examples of outcomes that can be examined in time out-of school programs include homework completion, responses to conflict, employment, sexual activity, civic leadership, and drug use.

Outcome evaluation will tell you:

- To what extent has the program achieved its goals?
- Is the current performance different from the past?
- Has the program been more successful than a comparable program?
- Which characteristics/activities are most related to success?
- What are the intended/unintended effects of the program?

Steps to address outcomes:

- Create realistic outcomes—focus on what the program realistically can accomplish
- Be specific—translate program goals into specific and measurable indicators
- Select evaluation design to fit your program—any desired behavioral change should be assessed
- Select methods for measurement—choose how to collect the data

What should be measured?

- Desired Outcomes often include changes in:
  - Knowledge—What people learned about a subject
  - Attitudes—How people feel about a subject

- Skills—How peoples' skills/abilities affect a problem by themselves (e.g., saying no to smoking)
- Behaviors—How people change their way of doings things (decrease in negative health habits or increase in positive health habits)

Determining Data Collection Methods

Before you spend any time or resources collecting data, be sure your community assessment plan adheres to these helpful standards:

- Feasible—Will the assessment be practical, realistic, and achievable? Is it doable?
- Useful—Will the amount and type of information you collect meet the needs of those who intend to use it? Will this information help to address the community public health needs you identified?
- Accurate—Will the assessment methodologies collect information that accurately reflects reality?
- Fair—Will the assessment be conducted with awareness of the rights of the people involved?
- Responsive—Is the assessment guided by the community needs, defined problems, goals, objectives, and assessment questions articulated by the partnership throughout the planning process?

There are a number of ways to collect data but there is no one single best way.

- Select methods of data collections
- Select data collections instruments
- Determine who is studied and when
- Select what method you will use:
  - Quantitative data are usually measured and expressed in the form of numbers or percentages. This data can answer the who, what, when, and where questions of an assessment.
  - Qualitative data is usually measured and expressed in the form of words, concepts, themes, or categories rather than numbers. Qualitative data is often used to gain a more in-depth understanding of a particular incident or phenomenon—they answer how or why something is occurring.
  - Mixed Method can be combined to collect both quantitative and qualitative data at one time. For example, focus group participants can be given a brief quantitative survey before or after the focus group, in addition to the qualitative discussion that would occur during the focus group.
  - Asset Mapping is an inventory of community health assets, such as available resources, services, facilities, community-based organizations and associations. Usually represented by geographically mapped data.

The decision about which approaches to use depends upon:

- What you need to know
- Where the data reside

- Resources and time available
- Complexity of the data to be collected
- Frequency of data collection.

The most commonly used methods in evaluation:

- Document analysis—Primarily quantitative but can also collect qualitative data in the form of documented narratives
- Surveys—Primarily quantitative but can also collect qualitative data through open-ended or free response questions
- Interviews—Primarily qualitative but can also collect quantitative data by numerically coding interview responses and/or observations
- Observations—Primarily qualitative but can also collect quantitative data by numerically coding observations.
- Focus groups—Primarily qualitative but can also collect quantitative data by numerically coding participant responses and/or observations.
- Case studies—Primarily qualitative but can also collect quantitative data by coding observations, using surveys and document analysis.

Gathering Data
Consider several ethical issues related to the collection and storing of data from human subjects when planning your evaluation.

- Informed consent—You should provide information to study participants about the purpose of the evaluation, how their responses will be used, and any possible consequences of their participation.
- Anonymity and confidentiality—These two terms are often used interchangeably, but they have different meanings. Make clear to respondents which term applies to them as part of informed consent.
  - *Anonymity* means you cannot identify respondents based on their responses. Anonymity makes follow-up difficult but can encourage respondents to be more honest in their responses.
  - *Confidentiality* means the investigator knows the identity of respondents but promises not to reveal it.

Data Security
Once collected, it is important to protect and secure data containing respondent identifiers in a locked file or room. Continue maintaining data security even after the study is complete or destroy your data by deleting or shredding it. Study Participant data that contains identifiers must be disposed of according to your Institutional Review Board (IRB).

Analyzing and Interpreting the Data—Justifying Conclusions
Data analysis and interpretation is the process of assigning meaning to the collected information and determining the conclusions, significance, and implications of the findings. The steps involved in data analysis are a function of the type of

information collected; however, returning to the purpose of the assessment and the assessment questions will provide a structure for the organization of the data and a focus for the analysis.

The analysis of numerical data (Quantitative) is represented in mathematical terms. The most common statistical terms include:

- Mean—The mean score represents a numerical average for a set of responses.
- Standard deviation—The standard deviation represents the distribution of the responses around the mean. It indicates the degree of consistency among the responses. The standard deviation, in conjunction with the mean, provides a better understanding of the data.
- Frequency distribution—The frequency distribution Indicates the frequency of each response. It provides additional information beyond the mean, since it allows for examining the level of consensus among the data.
- Higher levels of statistical analysis (e.g., t-test, factor analysis, regression, ANOVA) can be conducted on the data, but these are not frequently used in most program/project assessments.

The analysis of narrative (Qualitative) data is conducted by organizing the data into common themes or categories. It is often more difficult to interpret narrative data since it lacks the built-in structure found in numerical data. Initially, the narrative data appears to be a collection of random, unconnected statements. The assessment purpose and questions can help direct the focus of the data organization. The following strategies may also be helpful when analyzing narrative data.

Focus groups and Interviews:

- Read and organize the data from each question separately. This approach permits focusing on one question at a time (e.g., experiences with tutoring services, characteristics of tutor, student responsibility in the tutoring process).
- Group the comments by themes, topics, or categories. This approach allows for focusing on one area at a time (e.g., characteristics of tutor—level of preparation, knowledge of content area, availability).
- Documents—Code content and characteristics of documents into various categories (e.g., training manual—policies and procedures, communication, responsibilities).
- Observations—Code patterns from the focus of the observation (e.g., behavioral patterns, amount of time engaged/not engaged in activity, type of engagement, communication, interpersonal skills).
- The analysis of the data via statistical measures and/or narrative themes should provide answers to the assessment questions. Interpreting the analyzed data from the appropriate perspective allows for determination of the significance and implications of the assessment

Example of Program Evaluation—Data

Each funded program is required to collect several pieces of information about the type of activities, the number of persons served by the program, and characteristics

Table 5.1 Program reach

Client characteristic	Field	Reporting metric
Age	Date of birth (if not available, age at appointment)	Percent in each category on report OR *Mean, median, standard deviation
Race/ethnicity	Komen report categories	Percent in each category
Language	English versus other (type)	Percent non-English Speaking; Percent in each of the five top languages served
Screening habits	Never had Sporadic Regular	Percent in each
Location	County	Percent in counties in Komen report
Foreign born*	Yes/No	Percent foreign born
Date of last screening**	Define recommended screening test (mammogram, CBE, BSE, frequency?)	Percent screened within last year if over 40

Note Report Timeframe of each (year, quarter, etc.)
*Not required by funder but may be helpful in program planning
**Funder asks for an estimate of persons never screened, sporadically screened, and regularly screened. By collecting date of last screen from participants, you can categorize responses as follows: Never screened = No Date of Last Screening; >2 years = sporadic; Within 2 years = regular

of persons served by the program. Below we will show how these data can be used to answer the questions posed above. Table 5.1 (Program Reach) helps to gather and report data on the extent of reach by the program under evaluation; Table 5.2 (Program Adoption) helps to tabulate adoption statistics; and Table 5.3 (Program Implementation/Maintenance) provides data on the success of the program execution.

Reach

Report by the program REACH by Type of Service as outlined on the reporting spreadsheet (Prevention, Early Detection, Diagnosis, MRI, Biopsy, Treatment, Assistance Program; as well as persons lost to follow-***up)***

Adoption

See Table 5.2.

Table 5.2 Program adoption

Characteristics of setting	Field	Metric
Geography	Urban versus rural	Percent in each
Patient volume	Number of clients seen at facility/agency (per month, year)	Total number of patients served (not just navigated)
Nature of Services provided	Clinical versus Not (Yes/No)	Percent of each
If Clinical, type (primary, radiology, med onc, etc.)	Service type	Percent of each, if applicable
Services provided	CBE, mammography (type), ultrasound, MRI, biopsy	Percent of each, if applicable
Service capacity	Same day Wait time	Percent yes Mean, SD of wait times
Characteristics of navigators*	Age, gender, race/ethnicity, Language, foreign born qualifications Salary	Same as REACH + Qualifications (number years, experience, education, etc.) Salary (Mean, SD)
Program eligibility*	Describe any criteria	Percent who meet eligibility criteria/total patient volume
Program funding*	Competitive Grant Institution Endowment/Gift	Percent of total funding in each

Note Report Timeframe of each (year, quarter, etc.)
*Not required by funder but may be helpful in program planning

Implementation/Maintenance

See Table 5.3.

Effectiveness

There are three major categories of navigation activities (other than cost) toward proving effectiveness (Freund et al. 2008):

- Time to completion (from time to diagnosis resolution, or time to completion of therapy)
- Time to initiation of primary therapy (secondary—what is the quality of that care?)
- Patient-reported outcomes (satisfaction, quality of life, knowledge and self-efficacy)

Important: Collect dates for all activities. The best way to collect this type of information is to add it to forms or other sources of data you are already using,

Table 5.3 Program implementation and maintenance

Activity	Field	Metric
Total number of clients	Average caseload, daily/monthly	Client/navigator ratio
Type of contact	Letters sent Phone calls made	Total number of each
No show rates by type of appointment (screening or treatment) for navigators based in healthcare organizations*, **	Requires coordination with scheduling center to gather and analyze	Percent cancel, reschedule, no show, arrive
Outreach events	Name/describe audience and event or messages released	Number of events Estimated # in attendance or reached in message
Client contact*	Date of first encounter Date of closing meeting	Mean, median, SD of time interval
Type of barriers addressed*	Financial, attitudinal, transportation, patient focused comorbidity, system, interpersonal.	Percent in each category of barrier (identify most common)
Number of barriers addressed per client (Acuity)*	Sum up number of barriers/patient from checklist, or add a field for total number of barriers	Mean, median, standard deviation Percent with 1, 2, 3, etc. barriers
Education provided to client*, **	By disease type or barrier (yes/no)	Percent provided with education Of those provided, percent by type of education
Goals of treatment documented and discussed with patient**	By disease type (yes/no)	Percent of clients with a diagnosis who have goals of treatment documented and discussed, by disease type
Client self-reported confidence in adhering to plan**	Rating 1–5	Mean, median SD Report by different patient characteristics, such as described in REACH, or by number or type of barriers
Clients who stay within system for treatment (for navigators based in healthcare organization)*	Number diagnosed at facility Number who stay at facility for treatment	Ratio of diagnosed/stay for treatment
Number of referrals made (physical therapy, social work, etc.)*, **	Yes/No, by referral type	Percent referred, by disease type and referral type
Referral to clinical trials*, **	Yes/No	Percent referred
Client satisfaction with care**	Overall satisfaction rating 1–5	Mean, median, SD Report by different patient characteristics, such as

(continued)

Table 5.3 (continued)

Activity	Field	Metric
		described in REACH, or by number or type of barriers
Client satisfaction with navigator**	Overall satisfaction rating 1–5	Mean, median, SD Report by different patient characteristics, such as described in REACH, or by number or type of barriers

Note Report Timeframe of each (year, quarter, etc.)
*Not required by funder but may be helpful in program planning and proving impact
**Recommended by the Association of Community Cancer Centers

rather than add a new field to a database or a new form. Collecting timeliness data also allows the tracking of persons lost, because dates will be missing in corresponding fields. In order to capture TIMELINESS data, the following fields should be collected and tracked [3]:

- Date of abnormal screening test
- Date of abnormal test or symptom
- Stage at diagnosis
- Date of diagnosis (biopsy/pathology) or Date of resolution (no further activity needed)
- Date of notification of patient
- Date of initiation of primary therapy (by type—i.e., surgery, chemo, radiation)

Using these dates, you can report:

- Interval from screening test (or symptom) to diagnosis or resolution (mean, median, SD)
- Interval from diagnostic confirmation to patient notification
- Number with diagnostic resolution (% within 30, 60, 90 days of diagnosis)
- Interval from diagnostic confirmation to consultation with oncology specialist
- Interval from consultation to date of first treatment (primary therapy)
- Number with treatment initiation (% within 30, 60, 90 days)
- Number with abnormal screening test and no date of diagnosis or resolution (percent lost to follow-up from screening)*, **
- Number with date of diagnosis and no date of first treatment (percent lost to follow-up in treatment)*, **
- Percent of patients diagnosed at each stage (% with late diagnosis, over time) *, **
- *Required by funder
- **For navigators based in a healthcare institution, can only be reported for patients who receive care within your institution, so result may not be accurate —report limitations

To Compare or Not Compare, That is the Evaluation Question

Descriptive Information: Tabulating the information you gather using the metrics described above in RE-AIM will allow you to see a comprehensive picture, or description, of your program. By examining the proportions, means, and other summaries of the information, you can see patterns and describe the impact of your activities. You can answer questions described in the beginning of this section, such as, "Who are my clients and what are their needs? What are the benefits of my program?"

You can also group the information in ways that are meaningful. Perhaps you would like to examine the date of last screening among minority women in your program. Or, you would like to know the average age of those diagnosed at late stage. Descriptive information shown in the tables can be used in multiple combinations to better target resources and activities.

Making Comparisons: However, descriptive information does not provide a comparison. If you want to know if a change has occurred, you need to have two points in time to compare. This is commonly called a pre/post, or before/after, comparison. Instead of a before/after design, you may have thought about comparing your program to another program, or even what happens when there is no program. However, this type of comparison is not feasible to properly design by most programs. This is because the groups being compared must be virtually indistinguishable from each other with the exception of the program being delivered. Most service programs, unless they have specific research collaborations and dollars to support, cannot conduct this degree of evaluation toward proving effectiveness. However, it is possible to compare outcomes across time. You can also compare within categories to answer questions such as, "Is my program serving more women over versus under 50? Is my program serving more women from one county than another?" Also, it may be possible to compare your own program results OVER TIME to answer questions such as, "Is the number of clients served changing over time? Is the proportion of patients with early diagnosis improving over time?".

If you can report your program results over time, you should note the timeframe (between quarters, years, etc.) and also note any other relevant activities in your program that may have affected your conclusions. Did the facility get a new bus stop put in front? Did you add providers if located in a healthcare organization? Did the demographic or your clients' change? These are common sense, but can all affect interpretation of any comparisons you might make over time and should be noted in a general sense when commenting on your program effectiveness.

Defining Effectiveness: The Numbers Look Good, but How Do I Know the Program Made a Difference?

We all observed variation in a typical day. Sometimes it takes you 20 minutes to get to work, the next 30 day. Sometimes a bunch of bananas weighs 1 lb, sometimes more. If you want to know if the differences you observe are real or just "expected" variation, statistical analysis are used. Simple basic statistics calculators are available free on the Internet and can be used so long as a few basic steps are followed. Some examples are described below.

Comparing the Mean, Median, SD (Continuous factors)

Any factors described in RE-AIM that are measured and reported with a mean or average value can be compared using a t-test. However, there are a few precautions outlined in the example below.

EXAMPLE Question: Is my agency serving more people now than last year?

Comparing the Proportion (Percents, ratios)

Any factors described above in RE-AIM [4] that are measured and reported in counts, percents, or ratios can be compared using a Chi Square Test. The only limitation is that no one count can be below five or the numbers are too small for an adequate statistical comparison.

Example: Before the initiation of the navigation program, 60% of women diagnosed with breast cancer in our community were diagnosed with early stage disease. This was calculated based on observations collected between 2006 and 2008. The number of women served in this time period is 1000. After the program was funded in 2009, the proportion of women diagnosed with early stage disease increased to 71%. The total number of women served between 2009 and 2011 was 1200.

Step 1. Calculate the actual numbers, not just proportion, to enter into the statistical calculator. In this example, we converted 60% of 1000 to 600 and 71% of 1200 to 852.
Step 2. Using OpenEpi calculator, 2 X 2 Chi Square tab, this data was entered as shown below. As in our previous example, the p-value tells us whether or not the difference exceeds what is expected, and therefore is likely real. In this case, the p-value is 0.0001 or much smaller than 0.05. This means there is very little chance (much less than the usually accepted 5% chance) that this difference is due to expected variation. Therefore, the proportion of women diagnosed after program initiation is significantly higher AFTER the navigation than before.

What Else Should I Consider When Designing and Implementing an Evaluation Plan for My Program?

Regardless of how big or small the program, or the corresponding evaluation efforts, the evaluation plan should subscribe to the following recognized principles [5]:

1. Utility—it must be USEFUL; how will the results be used for one (or more) of the above-described purposes?
2. Feasibility—Can outcomes be measured? Does it cost more to measure the outcome than to provide navigation services? Will navigators be willing and able to provide the data?
3. Propriety—Is it ethical and fair to the patients, the navigators, and the providers to collect and report the information?

4. Accuracy—If all the above are yes, is what being collected an accurate way to measure the impact or outcome? Is what I am collecting the same as others, and/or based on a published method or tool? This includes using statistical tools described above—did you use the right test in the right way?

Dissemination—Ensure use and share lessons learned
Sharing the results of the program evaluation is an imperative step. This dissemination can take many forms but is an opportunity to share the successes and challenges of your program with others so they can try to replicate results or avoid the challenges. Dissemination can occur through formal academic means such as publication in journals or presentation at conferences. It can also occur informally through patient navigator networks (e.g., email newsletters). Informing others of your program will enhance future programs and may inform policies in order to improve future work.

Resources on Program Evaluation
Atkinson, A., Deaton, M., Travis, R., and Wessel, T. 1998. *The Virginia Effective Practices Project Programming and Evaluation Handbook. A Guide for Safe and Drug-free Schools and Communities Act Programs.* James Madison University and Virginia Department of Education

Bliss, M. J., Emshoff, J. G. 2002. *Workbook for Designing a Process Evaluation.* Atlanta, GA

https://www.researchgate.net/publication/237781138_Workbook_for_Designing_a_Process_Evaluation

Bond, S., Boyd, S., and Rapp, K. 1997. *Taking Stock: A Practical Guide to Evaluating Your Own Programs.* Horizon Research, Inc.

Center for Disease Control and Prevention. A Framework for Program Evaluation. Available at http://www.cdc.gov/eval/framework/index.htm

Center for Substance Abuse Prevention. 1998. *A Guide for Evaluating Prevention Effectiveness. Substance Abuse and Mental Health Services Administration Technical Report.*

Chinman M, Imm P, Wandersman A (2004). *Getting to Outcomes 2004: Promoting Accountability Through Methods and Tools for Planning, Implementation, and Evaluation.* Santa

Katz, Mira L., et al. "Barriers reported among patients with breast and cervical abnormalities in the patient navigation research program: Impact on timely care." *Women's Health Issues* 24.1 (2014): e155-e162

Komen Grant Applications. http://southflorida.info-komen.org/site/DocServer/2016-2017_South_Florida_Breast_Health_Navigation_and_Edu.pdf?docID=13548

Logic Models. http://djjr-courses.wikidot.com/ppol225-text:charts-and-diagrams-logic-models

Monica, CA: RAND Corporation, TR-TR101. Available at http://www.rand.org/publications/TR/TR101/.

References

1. Wholey JS, Hatry HP, Newcomer KE, editors. Handbook of practical program evaluation. 3rd ed. San Francisco: Jossey-Bass; 2010. ISBN 978-0-470-52247-9.
2. Advanced Methods in Delivery System Research—Planning, Executing, Analyzing, and Reporting Research on Delivery System Improvement. Content last reviewed July 2013. Agency for Healthcare Research and Quality, Rockville, MD. http://www.ahrq.gov/professionals/prevention-chronic-care/improve/coordination/webinar03/logicmodelsl.html.
3. Guadagnolo BA, Dohan D, Raich P. Metrics for evaluating patient navigation during cancer diagnosis and treatment. Cancer. 2011.
4. Re-Aim. Reach Effectiveness adoption implementation maintenance. http://www.re-aim.hnfe.vt.edu/about_re-aim/index.html. Virginia Polytechnic Institute and State University. 2016.
5. Patton M. Utilization-based evaluation. Beverly Hills: Sage Publications; 1986.

Chapter 6
Prevention and Early Detection Case Study: Patient Navigation in the Breast Health Program at Boston Medical Center

Molly McCoy, Sarah E. Caron and Tracy A. Battaglia

This chapter will describe the experience from the implementation of a Patient Navigation program within the Breast Health Center at Boston University Medical Center, an academic safety net institution serving a diverse urban population in Boston, Massachusetts. We first describe the development of the program, as a means to address observed disparities in the delivery of breast health services, and then share the evolution of the program as we refined the theoretical framework and scope of Patient Navigation to meet our community needs. The final section will describe the essential lessons learned to guide best practice implementation and evaluation of Patient Navigation as a model for reducing disparities in prevention and early detection in breast cancer.

M. McCoy (✉)
Section of General Internal Medicine, Women's Health Unit,
Boston Medical Center, Boston University, 801 Massachusetts Avenue, Boston,
MA 02119, USA
e-mail: mollymcc@pcom.edu

S.E. Caron
Section of General Internal Medicine, Women's Health Unit, Department
of Medicine, Boston Medical Center, Boston University School of Medicine,
801 Massachusetts Ave, First Floor, Boston, MA 02118, USA
e-mail: sarahcaron14@gmail.com

T.A. Battaglia
Department of Medicine, Boston Medical Center, 801 Massachusetts Ave,
Crosstown Building, 1st Floor, Boston, MA 02118, USA
e-mail: tracy.battaglia@bmc.org

E.A. Calhoun and A. Esparza (eds.), *Patient Navigation*,
DOI 10.1007/978-1-4939-6979-1_6

Why Start a Program?

The Breast Health Center at Boston Medical Center (the teaching hospital of Boston University School of Medicine and the largest safety net institution in New England) was created in 1989 through collaboration between the Women's Health Unit (a primary care clinic and research unit), Surgical and Medical Oncology, and Breast Imaging. In addition to providing one-stop shopping for all breast health needs, it is a unique model of specially trained internists and surgeons offering comprehensive breast diagnostic services [1]. Since its inception, the breast health program has provided diagnostic breast health Patient Navigation services to over 20,000 women, most of whom are low-income and/or racial/ethnic minorities. Those served are diverse and reflective of the urban population seeking care at an inner city safety net institution. The majority of women seeking care are of minority race or ethnicity, 33% Black, 30% Hispanic, 5% Asian. One-third require a language interpreter during their visit, and over half have publicly funded or no health insurance at the time of their referral. About half of referrals come from a network of over 15 affiliated community health centers, and the other half from practices within the Medical Center campus clinical practice sites including primary care, specialty services and the Emergency Department. The two most frequent reasons for referral triaged to internists are abnormal breast exam (54%) and breast pain (26%), followed by family history of breast cancer, abnormal imaging, and nipple discharge.

In the year 2000, the providers in the Breast Health Center recognized the presence of a high rate of missed appointments. During any given clinical session nearly half of all scheduled patients did not arrive for their clinical evaluation. Data at the time showed that women referred by a community health center and women of African descent were more likely to miss an appointment. Most concerning was that other local data also found that women from these inner city communities had lower rates of mammography, higher rates of breast cancer, and more advanced stages of cancer at diagnosis [2–4]. Thus, the Avon Foundation for Women generously supported the Avon Breast Health Initiative targeting women challenged by language, cultural, and economic barriers. The program was conceived as a clinical services initiative to enhance the quality of care for these at-risk women in need of diagnostic breast cancer care.

Identifying the Problem

A comprehensive needs assessment was conducted in order to provide an evidence-base for identifying the problem and finding a solution [5]. Twenty patients who had missed their appointment were contacted and asked only about the reason for not keeping their appointment and their opinions on what could be done to reduce the missed appointment rates. One-on-one, face-to-face, open-ended interviews were conducted with stakeholders from the Breast Health Center including support staff, physicians (specialty providers and referring providers from community health centers), interpreters, and 14 patients (eight established and six new). Full length interviews consisted of four to seven open ended questions and lasted between 15–30 min. All interviews were given between 6/30/01-8/3/01 by a trained summer research intern who had prior knowledge of the program.

Major Findings and Themes

There were a few major themes that emerged from repeated mention by all of the stakeholders. These common themes were lack of resources, poor communication, lack of coordination of services including radiology, and exceptional quality of care (Table 6.1).

From these findings, it was clear that our practice was in need of more resources for improving clinic efficiency, better communication between each facet of care and within the clinic, and increased coordination of care across the board. The information gained from the needs assessment was then used to construct a formal action plan to improve care delivery within the Breast Health Center. The consensus of providers from these findings was a need for additional resources to target care coordination that focuses on the unique needs of the multiple disciplines and culturally diverse patient population.

Feasibility: Pilot Patient Navigation

An examination of the literature revealed that care management was a promising approach to target an at-risk population by providing care coordination that addresses the unique sociocultural issue that was uncovered in the needs assessment. Patient Navigation, an emerging model of care coordination encompassing both community-based outreach and coordination activities, seeks to address known barriers to the delivery of high-quality cancer care [2, 6–8]. Thus, a Patient Navigation Pilot Intervention project was developed in order to assess the feasibility of Patient Navigation in the Breast Health Center to address the identified needs.

A pre/post pilot study was designed as a quality improvement project [9]. The main objective of the intervention was to improve the rate of timely diagnostic follow-up, and to identify characteristics of patients who are most at risk of being lost to follow-up. The major outcome was "timely follow-up" (yes/no), defined as arrival to an appointment within 120 days of originally scheduled appointment [10–12].

From January–June 2000, patients 18 years or older who were referred to the Breast Health Center were included in the pre-intervention group. No changes to existing referral, scheduling, or reminder systems were made during this time.

Table 6.1 Needs assessment findings

Theme	Staff	Interpreters	Referring providers	Internal providers	Patients
Lack of resources					
Needs					
More space (waiting area, exam rooms, offices)	X				
More staff (administrative, medical assistant)	X				
A tracking system (to track patients)	X				
Inefficiencies					
Inefficiencies leading to long wait times					X
Insufficient time booked for new patients		X			
Poor communication					
Intercommunication issues	X	X	X	X	X
Wait times, resulting in missing other appointments					X
Hard to cancel appointments due to busy phone					X
Unaware of scheduled appointments					X
Explanation why interpreter left appointments early		X			
Not enough time to address sociocultural issues		X			
Lack of results communication from radiology				X	
Lack of coordination of services					
New staff are unaware of key stakeholder roles	X			X	
Patient flow issues	X			X	
Lack of protocols and guidelines	X				
Scope of work of Interpreters not clear to staff		X			
Training needed for making outside referrals	X				
Long wait times for breast imaging services				X	
Reporting results to patient before provider	X				
Poor communication of patient follow-up plan	X				
Poor communication about films and loss of films	X				
Quality of clinical care					
High-quality patient care delivery		X	X		X

Administrative staff would attempt telephone contact with patients to remind them of appointments but did not receive any clinical oversight. November 2001 began the post, or intervention, period. Again, all 18 years and over patients referred to the Breast Health Center were included in the intervention group and received navigation services.

One of the Breast Health Center's Medical Assistants, a member of the target community with 10 years experience working in the medical practice, was hired and trained as a Patient Navigator. Guided by the principles of care management [13], and under the supervision of two physician providers, four key Patient Navigator activities were defined:

1. Case identification
2. Identification of individual barriers to care
3. Implementation of a care plan
4. Tracking through completion

The navigator was trained on these principles with a particular focus on cultural competency and systematically identifying barriers to care at the individual patient level. Written triage and follow-up protocols were developed for the navigator's use. The navigator contacted all patients referred for diagnostic evaluation one week before their scheduled visit by telephone to confirm appointments, provide information about the visit, and elicit any individual barriers to attending the appointment. Interpreters were used for non-English speaking women. The navigator then utilized available resources to help patients address their barriers, for example, scheduling appropriate interpreters for appointments. Advocating for patients with breast abnormalities and referring patients to providers and other specialty sites (radiology, surgery, and pathology) were also key activities of the navigator. With regular oversight from the study coordinator, the navigator would track information on patient demographics, referral information, diagnostic evaluation, and outcomes.

In total, 1332 women were included in the study, 314 were pre-intervention and 1018 were intervention. The majority were under 65 years old, of minority race (40% Black, 14% Hispanic, and 4% Asian), and had no insurance or public insurance (68%). Fifteen percent required a language interpreter during their visit. Overall, 64% of subjects had timely follow-up during the pre-intervention period compared with 78% during the intervention ($p < 0.001$, unadjusted OR: 2.0 [95% CI 1.5, 2.6]). When controlling for age, race, insurance status, reason for referral, and source of referral, women in the intervention group had a 39% increased chance of having timely follow-up (OR = 1.39 [95% CI 1.01–1.91]). While all women benefited from navigation services, we did find that women who were referred from community health centers did worse than those referred from hospital-based practices (OR 1.4, 95% CI 1.0–2.0).

Expansion of Patient Navigation Program

Upon demonstration of these initial benefits of Patient Navigation into the clinical services program, we were interested in the potential advantage of introducing navigation into other settings, specifically expanding navigation across the cancer care spectrum and into the community health centers' primary care services, in order to answer the following questions:

(1) *Would navigation be an effective means to improve cancer screening rates, or improve access to timely cancer treatment?*
(2) *Would navigation out in the community allow us to reach the most vulnerable populations?*

Expansion to Breast Cancer Screening

Lower mammography screening rates among minority and low-income women are well-known contributors to increased morbidity and mortality from breast cancer. We sought to implement a breast cancer screening Patient Navigation program to measure the effect of navigation on increasing adherence rates to biennial screening mammography among women engaged in primary care at Boston Medical Center [14]. To perform this task, we designed a quality improvement initiative that initially randomized at the level of the primary care provider, such that half of the patients in the practice, per provider, received Patient Navigation (intervention group), while the other half received usual care (control group), allowing for a rigorous evaluation. After the initial intervention period, all control subjects still in need of mammography received navigation services.

Patients assigned to navigation whose last mammogram was more than 18 months prior received a combination of telephone calls and reminder letters from the navigators. Navigators were integrated into primary care teams and interacted with patients, providers, and radiology directly to coordinate care. Navigators used an electronic report to track subjects. Adherence rates to biennial mammography were assessed at baseline and post-Patient Navigation intervention.

A total of 3865 women participated in the study, with 1817 assigned to Patient Navigation services and 2078 assigned to usual care serving as the controls. Mean age was 60 years, 71% were racial/ethnic minorities, 23% were non-English speaking, and 63% had public or no health insurance. Baseline assessment of adherence rates showed no difference between those in control and intervention groups (78%, respectively, $p = 0.55$). After the 9-month intervention, mammography adherence was higher in the intervention group (87% vs. 76%, respectively, $p < 0.001$). All racial/ethnic and insurance groups demonstrated higher adherence in the intervention group, except among Hispanic women, who demonstrated high rates in both intervention and control groups (85 and 83%, respectively).

These clinic-based studies provided rigorous evidence of the benefit that Patient Navigation has across the early part of the *cancer care continuum,* and set the stage for the next study which included navigation among those diagnosed with cancer.

Extension to Community Health Centers

As part of an existing collaboration with the Boston Health Net, a partnership between Boston Medical Center, and 15 Affiliated Community Health Centers, a Patient Navigation Community Advisory Panel was developed to guide the implementation study of navigation in the federally qualified community health centers in Boston. There was an alignment of priorities around the need to improve the coordination of cancer care services from screening through treatment for both breast and cervical cancer cases in the community. It was hypothesized that these women would benefit from additional support by someone from within their own community who knew the health system as well as the local culturally specific challenges in accessing care.

To test this hypothesis, the research team applied for and received funding from the National Cancer Institute's Center to Reduce Cancer Health Disparities to be part of the national Patient Navigation Research Program [4]. Following Community-Based Participatory Research (CBPR) principles, the study was designed in collaboration with community partners including the six Federally Qualified Community Health Centers sites affiliated with Boston Medical Center. The Community Advisory Board guided the study design and planning.

A quasi-experimental study with strategic allocation was implemented. The study looked at the impact of a Patient Navigator on the time to diagnosis for women with either a breast or cervical cancer screening abnormality. The Boston program was designed as a clinical effectiveness study of Patient Navigation as a new standard of care, where all patients with screening abnormalities were included into the trial and thus the Boston University Institutional Review Board approved the study with a waiver of written informed consent. Each health center was assigned a navigation site for either abnormal breast or cervical cancer screening and a control for the other condition (Fig. 6.1). The major benefit of this design was that each participating health center had the benefit of an intervention, while still ensuring the scientific rigor of the study by having clear, non-contaminated, continuous control groups.

The patients served by each health center are reflective of the local neighborhood and are unique to each health center. While the majority of patients are vulnerable in terms of low income, having public or no insurance, and low educational attainment, they varied center to center by race/ethnicity, language needs, and immigration status. For example, one partnering center had a large Vietnamese and Hispanic population, another mostly Black, nonimmigrant population, and a third served a large recently immigrant Albanian population. Over 4000 women

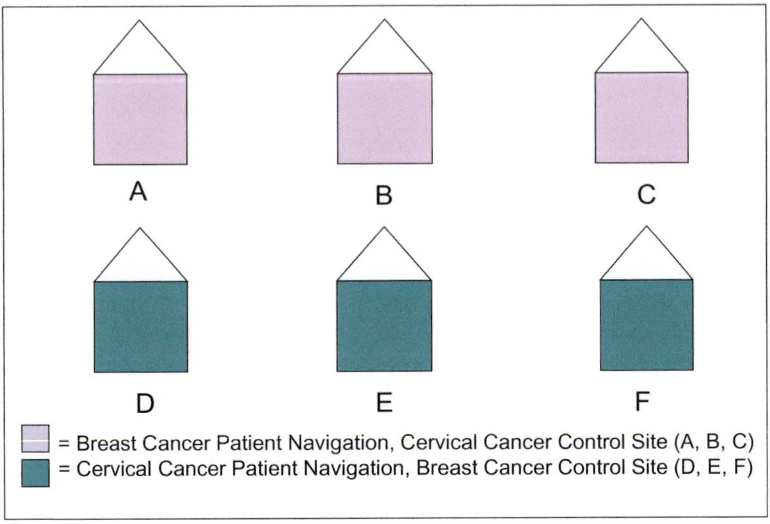

Fig. 6.1 Intervention and control site designation

participated in this study. Initial analyses document a benefit of Patient Navigation on timely diagnosis [15].

Theoretical Framework: An Evolving Model

Figure 6.2 below depicts the complex nature of cancer health disparities. Our model of Patient Navigation was designed to address those modifiable factors in the figure: patient, provider, and system barriers to accessing care across the continuum of care.

Our theory posits that a culturally competent community member trained to understand and interact with the health system would successfully navigate vulnerable patients into and through recommended care. To accomplish this, all of our navigation programs were modeled after the four principles of care management [13]. Again, these are:

1. Case Identification
2. Identification of individual barriers to care
3. Implementation of a care plan
4. Tracking through completion

These principles guide the entire Patient Navigation program, in addition to guiding each patient-navigator interaction. The four principles highlight the need for identifying those at risk for poor outcomes and then following them over time to ensure they remain compliant throughout their continuum of care, as well as the need for a patient-centered approach by identifying barriers that are unique to that

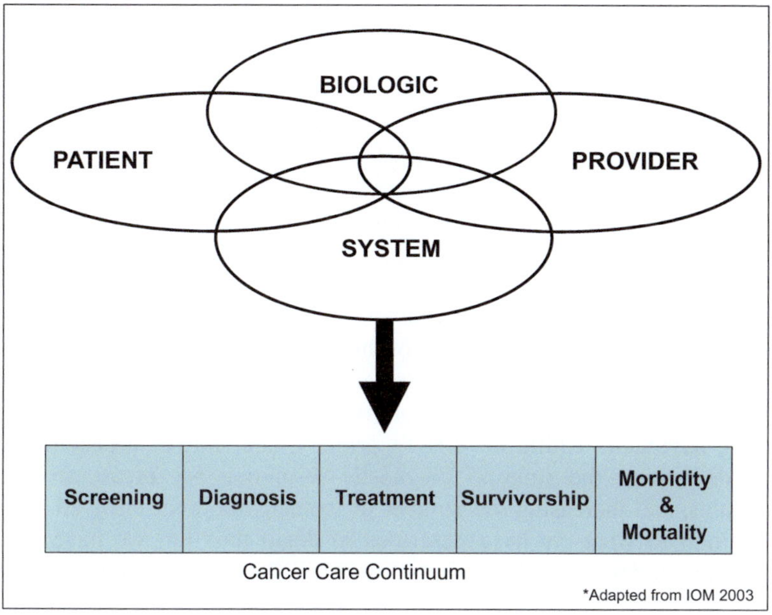

Fig. 6.2 Cancer care continuum

Table 6.2 Principles of care management applied

Principle	Navigator	Navigation team
Case identification	Navigator gets "flagged" within the EMR on an abnormal mammogram for all patients of Dr Smith's	Weekly reports of all missed diagnostic appointments are automatically generated
Identification of individual barriers to care	Navigator asks patients about potential barriers when scheduling, such as "do you need childcare?" and listens to the patient to identify issues such as fear or not understanding	Schedulers trained to ask each patient if they would like an interpreter present during their appointment, and booking the interpreter when appointment is made
Implementation of a care plan	Navigator confirms with Dr. Smith what follow-up appointments Patient A will need	Standardized protocols with time components for follow-up (e.g., BIRADS 3—follow-up mammogram scheduled 6–7 months)
Tracking through completion	Navigator calls each patient to remind them of appointments, and if they have missed an appointment to find out why and to reschedule them	Monthly, automated reports of all clinic patients who have had an abnormal mammogram and what their follow-up status is

patient. Table 6.2 provides some examples of how each principle is implemented by the Navigator for a particular patient, and how systems are put in place by the entire team for each principle.

Evolving Model

As a clinical and research unit, we have truly embraced navigation and see the benefit of having a system of navigation, as well as a navigator, as part of the care delivery team. As described here and depicted in Fig. 6.3, our model continuously evolves in response to our evaluation data. We started navigation based within the hospital for women with abnormal breast findings as a quality improvement project. When it showed success in increasing patients' follow-up, we looked to see who were benefiting the least [9].

Women referred from the CHCs have lower rates of follow-up compared to those who received their primary care at one of the hospital-based practices. Our national project grew out of a partnership with six community health centers to address these disparities, and to provide more rigorous Patient Navigation evaluation data. Integrating navigators within the CHC's primary care showed a benefit for these women, decreasing the time to diagnostic resolution for breast and cervical abnormalities, and increasing the number of women who ever resolved [15].

In addition to what we have described in detail thus far, we have expanded navigation in other ways, both in terms of the clinical site where navigators are team members and in the type of navigation services provided.

Navigation within the breast health center continues to help patients with abnormal screenings get the diagnostic care and treatment they need. We have expanded their role to include outreach to women who receive primary care at our hospital and who are >18 months overdue for their screening mammograms [14]. Navigators work to schedule mammogram appointments for these non-adherent patients. Recently, we expanded this effort to include patients who receive care at our Resident Clinics [16]. Navigators have also become an integral part of our overall Cancer Care team here at BMC. Oncology now utilizes five navigators to insure all cancer patients receiving care here at BMC get to their appointments, and have the support and resources they need to complete their treatment plans. There is also a team of clinical trial nurse navigators whose goal is to screen, educate, and recruit patients to cancer clinical trials available here.

Our data from the Patient Navigation Research Program breast subjects found that navigation did not have a benefit before 60 days, suggesting that there are patients who will get in for needed care quickly, with or without a navigator's assistance. However, after 60 days, having a navigator significantly benefits women. We hypothesize that it is patients who already have initial delays that will

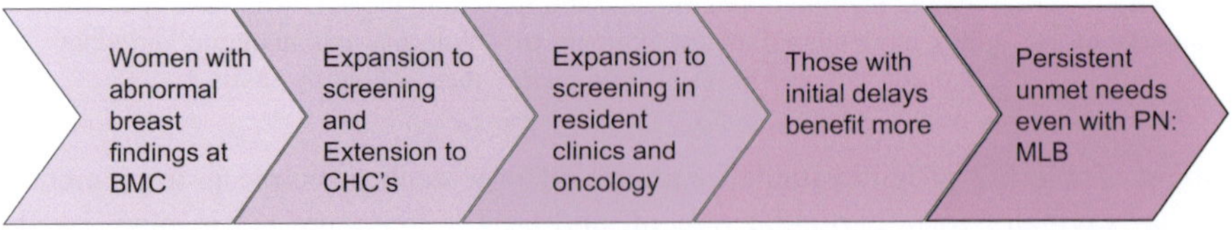

Fig. 6.3 Evolving Patient Navigation model

benefit more from Patient Navigation and testing models of navigation initiated after the first missed appointment or other delay that triggers a navigator to step in might be a more logical approach when faced with limited resources. Targeting populations which might benefit most from Patient Navigation is important to making Patient Navigation a cost-effective intervention, suggesting the need for ongoing comparative effectiveness research to identify best practices.

Finally, we have learned that the type of barriers and the ability of a navigator to address those barriers impacts the time it takes to get to diagnostic resolution. We also know that there are barriers that Patient Navigators just do not have resources to address, or are not able to identify, and therefore cannot address. We are currently collaborating with the Medical Legal Partnership | Boston, a legal advocacy program that seeks to address low-income patient concerns with legal solutions. We will test standard Patient Navigation compared to navigation enhanced by Medical Legal Partnership in a cancer population.

We offer the following general concepts to provide a working definition for Patient Navigation and the framework for others interested in adopting a similar framework [17]:

- Patient Navigation is a model of care that aims to reduce an existing health disparity as defined in a particular community.
- Patient Navigation addresses a patient's individual barriers to care by linking them to existing local and regional resources, not by creating new resources or services.
- Patient Navigation is not just a Patient Navigator; navigation requires a team approach: administrators to champion the program, supervisors to provide clinical and administrative support, *and* Patient Navigators with a defined role within the healthcare team.

These concepts have guided us as we put Patient Navigation into operation within our own institution and community. Although variations in the definition of Patient Navigation exist, we found that Patient Navigation is generally defined as a *barrier-focused intervention* (in this case, for cancer care) with seven common characteristics:

1. Navigation is provided to individual patients for a defined episode of care (e.g., through the evaluation of an abnormal screening test)
2. Navigation targets a defined set of health services that are required to complete an episode of care
3. Navigation has a defined endpoint when the provision of services is complete (e.g., patient achieves diagnostic resolution after a screening abnormality)
4. Navigation serves to bridge gaps in the existing healthcare system for individual patients
5. Navigation systems require coordination among members of the health services team

6. Navigation services focus on the identification and reduction of individual patient level barriers to accessing and completing care
7. Navigation aims to reduce delays in accessing the continuum of care services, with an emphasis on timeliness of diagnosis and treatment and a reduction in the number of patients lost to follow-up

Patient Navigator Skills and Scope of Work

Our group performed a qualitative study to develop a structured protocol for observing Patient Navigators at work, describing and characterizing specific activities related to their goals [18]. Over 130 h of observation of navigators across 18 programs was used to characterize the work of Patient Navigators and offers a tool for monitoring and evaluating what navigators do.

They found that navigator actions across a wide variety of settings can be categorized in a matrix with two dimensions. One dimension categorizes the individuals and organizational entities with whom the navigator interacts; the other characterizes the types of tasks carried out by the navigators in support of their patients. Use of this protocol will enable researchers to systematically characterize and compare navigator activities within and across different programs.

Six Patterns of Patient Navigation Action

Six patterns of Patient Navigation actions were identified during the group's observations. These are:

1. **Direct patient-focused** Primarily direct interaction with patients
2. **Network-focused** Little interaction with patients; facilitating care with supports, support services
3. **Support services-focused** Develops and maintains relationships with supports
4. **Indirect patient-focused** Indirect interaction with patients (e.g., messaging); little interaction with providers, staff, supports
5. **Patient and network-focused** Like pattern 4, plus frequent facilitating care with providers, clinic staff, and supports
6. **Working with medical records** Low rate of interaction with patients

Researchers found discrete patterns of navigators' activities that may vary by local context:

- Design of navigators' job
- Location of navigation
- Organization

- Workflow
- Physical placement of navigator
- Balance of navigation and other responsibilities

Standard Work of Patient Navigators

After evolution of the theoretical framework and supported by direct observation of navigators in the field [18], we have developed a structure for Patient Navigation activities (See Figs. 6.4 and 6.5). We categorize Patient Navigation activities into four major domains of work. Activities that occur in each domain are reflective of our founding principles (1) Case Identification, (2) Identification of individual barriers to care, (3) Implementation of a care plan, and (4) Tracking through completion.

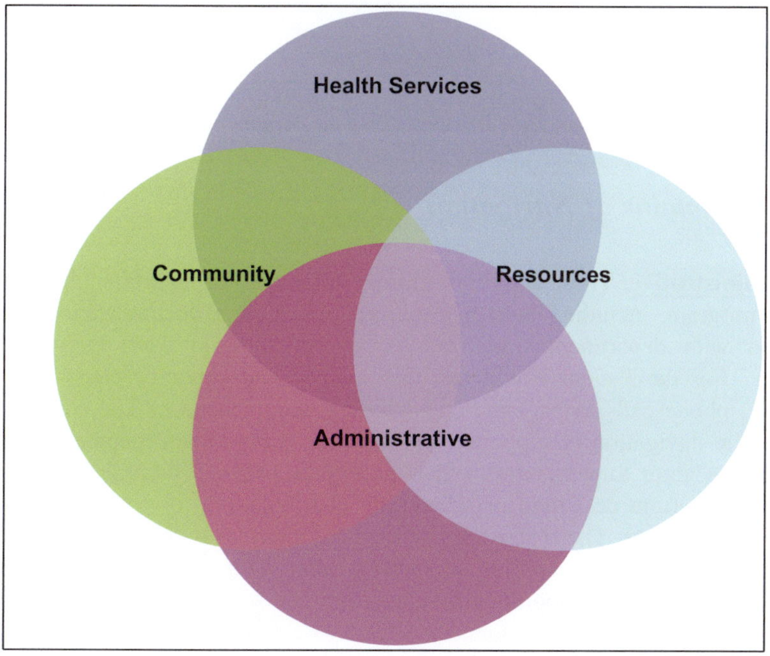

Fig. 6.4 Major domains of Patient Navigation activities

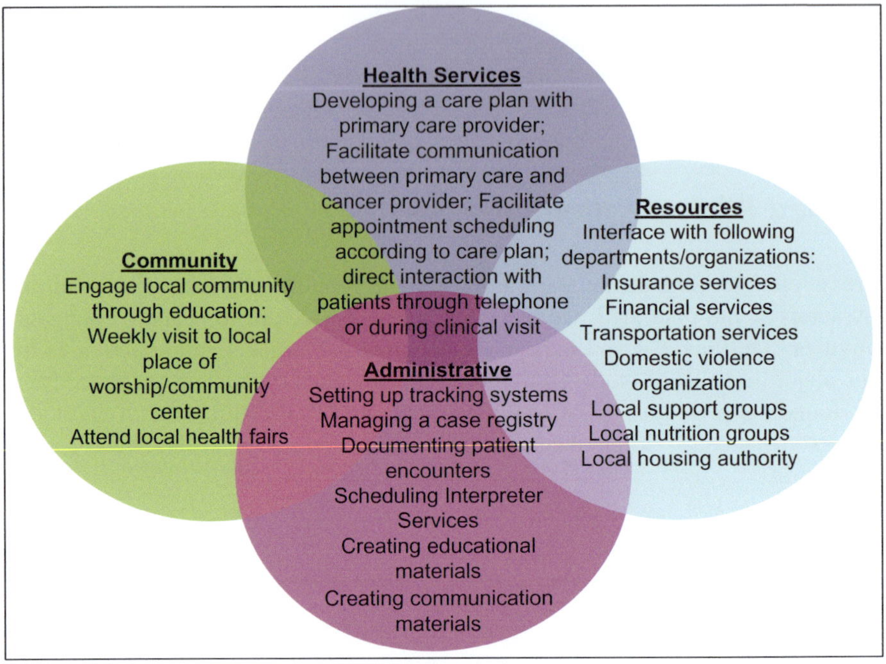

Fig. 6.5 Type of Patient Navigator activities across the domains

Major Domains of Navigation

Administrative: These activities address organizational and financial allocation of the program, including human resources, scheduling, documentation, communication with departments/organizations, coordination of care, budgeting, and funding. For the Patient Navigator, this includes all paper or electronic record keeping, phone calls to patients, and tracking documentation. The administrative side of the navigation is supported by other navigation team members, including Patient Navigator Supervisor(s), other leadership staff and administrative support staff (such as front desk staff or scheduling coordinators).

Health Services: These activities address the interface with health care delivery, including case-finding, tracking, communication with health services staff and providers, facilitating appointment scheduling for screening, diagnostics, and/or treatment. For Patient Navigators, this involves activities related to patients being navigated into and throughout their care. This part of the navigation team may include medical assistants, nurses, and physicians from multiple departments or clinics. These team members work with and support Patient Navigators and Patient Navigators work to keep the rest of the care team informed about patient needs.

Resources: These activities include finding and developing partnerships with internal and external programs and organizations that may allow the navigator to address barriers that hinder patients' ability to attain health services. Some examples include: departments of transportation, social work, employment services, insurance companies, food pantries, and interpretation services. The Patient Navigator actively seeks out resources within and outside the program to meet the needs of their patients.

Community: These activities occur in community settings and are intended to reach out to the target population served by the program. "Community" means the people the Patient Navigator serves, the neighborhoods their patients come from, and the different cultures found among these groups.

Training navigators to implement activities across these domains requires training of the navigator, their supervisor and even the healthcare system within which they work. Integrating the navigator into the healthcare team is a critical first step. Training navigators should be guided by core competencies, yet there is not yet general agreement about what they should be. Our program has concentrated on the following core skills [17]: (1) general organization and time management, (2) barrier identification, (3) resource identification and utilization, and (4) cultural responsiveness and sensitivity.

The following case study should help to frame how Patient Navigators interact with patients using all of these core competencies with the principles of navigation in mind.

Case Study: Standard Work of Patient Navigators

Cassandra, a 27-year-old woman new to the community the Patient Navigator serves, had never been to see a doctor in the United States. Cassandra had also never had a gynecological Pap test in her life. The Patient Navigator met her at the community center where she does outreach work to find people who might benefit from navigation, increase health awareness, and spread the word about the Patient Navigation Program which provides screening for cervical and breast cancer. After talking with Cassandra for a few minutes, the Patient Navigator encouraged her to make an appointment at the local community health center. The Patient Navigator asked Cassandra if there was a reason she had not been to see a doctor. Cassandra said that she did not feel sick. Cassandra said she did not really know where to go because she had only moved to that neighborhood a year ago. She said she also was not sure how to make an appointment because she does not know very much English. The Patient Navigator knew right away what to do, because she listened to Cassandra to try to understand why she was not getting health care. She assured Cassandra that she could make an appointment for her and arrange to have a medical interpreter during the visit so that communication would not be a problem. The Patient Navigator also told Cassandra that it was a good idea to get a physical exam just to check on things even if she was not feeling sick. She told Cassandra that it will be comforting to know that she is in good health after she gets the overdue Pap Test. Cassandra agreed that this sounded like the right thing to do and the Patient Navigator helped her make an appointment.

The Patient Navigator checked Cassandra's medical record to see what happened at the visit because it occurred on a day she was off. She read that the provider had wanted to do a Pap test, but it was noted that Cassandra had her period and the procedure could not be completed. The next note said that Cassandra had been told to reschedule for the following week. The Patient Navigator found that no other appointments had been booked. She called Cassandra to see what was up, but got no answer and had to leave a message. She tried calling three more times over the next 2 weeks and could not get in contact with Cassandra.

Weeks later, back at her outreach post at the community center where she does screenings, Cassandra approached the Patient Navigator. The Patient Navigator asked how everything was going and why she had not returned any of her phone calls. Cassandra admitted that she was nervous about the Pap test procedure and did not want it. She said that her friend told her it was weird and painful. The Patient Navigator comforted her, saying that many women are nervous about getting Pap tests. She told Cassandra that it is not the most comfortable procedure, but it can be a life saving one.

Cassandra told the Patient Navigator that in addition to her being nervous, the interpreter had not shown up for her visit. Without an interpreter, Cassandra was confused about what the provider was saying. The Patient Navigator told her that this time, she would go with her to the appointment and make sure a medical interpreter was there. This was enough to convince Cassandra to go and get the Pap test.

Effect of Patient Navigation: Tracking Progress and Outcomes

The lack of comparable metrics to evaluate prevention and early detection Patient Navigation programs impeded the ability to identify best practices. Commonly used measures to evaluate navigation programs fall into several categories, as defined by the corresponding goal:

(1) <u>Clinical outcome measures</u> evaluate the impact of navigation on health outcomes
(2) <u>Process measures</u> evaluate the impact of navigation on the delivery of health care services
(3) <u>Patient-reported outcome measures</u> evaluate the impact of navigation from the patient's perspective

The Prevention and Early Detection Workgroup of the Patient Navigation Leadership Summit was charged with making recommendations for common clinical outcome metrics specific to the prevention and early detection phase of the cancer care continuum. Recommendations for researchers and program evaluators included the following:

1. Clearly document key program characteristics
2. Use a set of core data elements to form the basis of your reported metrics
3. Prioritize data collection using methods with the least amount of bias

If navigation programs explicitly state the context of their evaluation and choose from among the common set of data elements, meaningful comparisons among existing programs should be feasible [19]. Examples of recommended outcome metrics for prevention and early detection navigation programs are listed in Table 6.3 [19].

Other outcomes to consider, sometimes called *intermediate outcomes*, can also be process measures. For the breast health program at Boston Medical Center, we monitor monthly metrics reports to assess navigation process measures in real time. Since navigation contact is initially conducted via telephone outreach, we monitor the outcome of the navigator telephone calls to assess whether the mode of contact is having its intended effect, namely to show up for their scheduled diagnostic appointment. These monthly charts allow us to monitor how alternations in our protocols are impacting care.

The next two figures detail the navigator-patient contact rate. The first (Fig. 6.6) tracks the type of contacts being made with patients, such as direct contact (speaking with patient in person or on the telephone) or indirect contact (leaving a voicemail or speaking with a member of the patient's household). The 'Other' category denotes an unable to reach category, which includes inability to leave a voicemail due to busy signal, no answer, or disconnected telephone line. The second figure (Fig. 6.7) graphs the show rate for each type of contact, allowing us

Table 6.3 Common measures by metric type

	Clinical measures	Process measures
Screening metrics	– # of each BIRADS – # of cancer diagnoses – Stage at diagnosis	– Receipt of screening test – Adherence to recommended screening – Receipt of next scheduled screening test – Barriers to screening test – Maintenance screening behavior – Timely adherence to diagnostic resolution – Number of kept appointments
Diagnostic metrics	– Receipt of diagnostic resolution – Stage at diagnosis	– Timely adherence to diagnostic resolution – Barriers to diagnostic resolution – Number of kept appointments

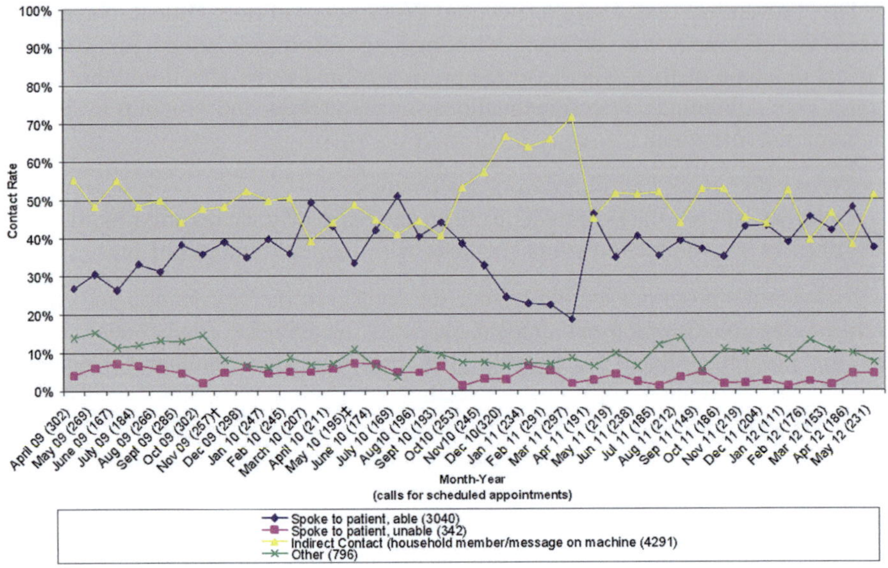

Fig. 6.6 Monthly navigator contact type rate

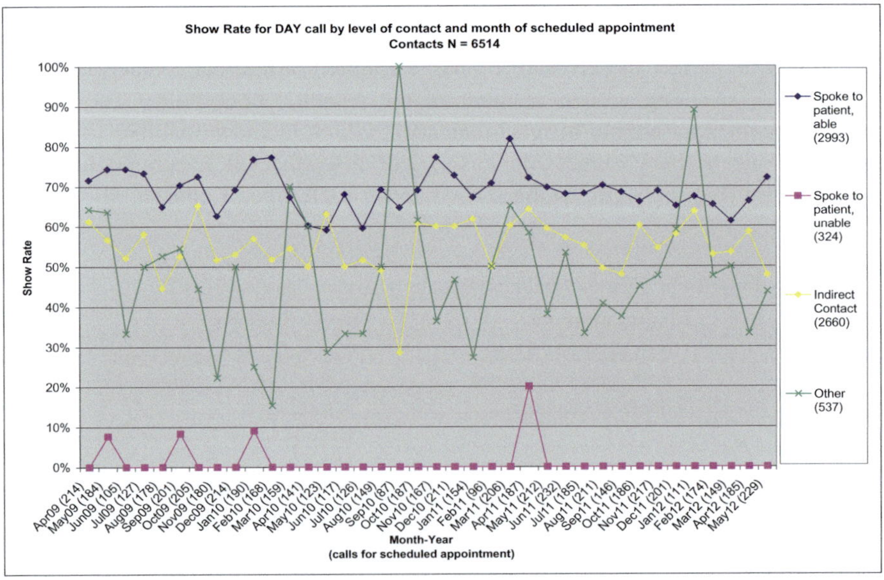

Fig. 6.7 Show rate by navigator contact type

to visualize what type of contact is most likely to result in attendance of a scheduled appointment.

In a recent study by Dr. Andrea Kronman, one of our Breast Health Center providers, it was found that for our population, patients who received direct contact from their navigator had three times the odds of completing their appointments compared to those with no contact (aOR 3.0, 95% CI 2.3, 4.0) [20].

Experience suggests that using process measures which capture the daily activities of navigators may be used to evaluate program delivery and its impact on appointment adherence. Furthermore, ongoing monitoring of these measures allows for practice adjustments to be made when established protocols fall short of delivering the highest quality care to all patients. Kronman et al. demonstrated that longitudinally tracking a process measure (contact type rate) and an intermediate outcome (appointment completion) could inform clinical protocols that increase the effectiveness of our navigator program.

It is important to remember that although better clinical outcomes is the ultimate goal, process measures and intermediate outcomes affect clinical outcomes, and should not be neglected.

Finally, with the increasing focus on providing patient-centered care, patient reported outcomes are integral to estimating the patient level effect of Patient Navigation. One common approach is assessing patient satisfaction through conducting surveys. Jean-Pierre et al. [21] validated the Patient Satisfaction with Interpersonal Relationship with Navigator (PSN-I), a measure for patients undergoing diagnostic and/or therapeutic cancer care [21]. They administered the PSN-1 to 783 patients from the nine different Patient Navigation Research Program sites and evaluated the structure and internal consistency, and looked at divergence and convergence of the PSN-I with the Patient Satisfaction with Cancer-related Care (PSCC), the Rapid Estimate of Adult Literacy in Medicine (REALM) Long Form, and patients' demographics. They found a coherent set of items that explicates 76.6% of the variance in PSN-I. Reliability assessment revealed high internal consistency (α ranging from 0.95 to 0.96). The PSN-I had good face validity as well as convergent and divergent validities as indicated by moderate correlations with score on the PSCC (all $p < 0.0001$) and nonsignificant correlations with primary language, marital status, and scores on the REALM Long Form (all $p > 0.05$). The group concluded that the PSN-I is a valid and suitable measure of satisfaction with a Patient Navigator for the present sample.

References

1. Battaglia TA, Howard MB, Kavanah M, et al. The addition of internists to a breast health program. Breast J. 2012;18(1):58–64.
2. Dohan D, Schrag D. Using navigators to improve care of underserved patients: current practices and approaches. Cancer. 2005;104(4):848–55.
3. Clegg LX, Reichman ME, Miller BA, et al. Impact of socioeconomic status on cancer incidence and stage at diagnosis: selected findings from the surveillance, epidemiology, and

end results: National longitudinal mortality study. Cancer Causes Control. 2009;20(4): 417–35.

4. Freund KM, Battaglia TA, Calhoun E, et al. National cancer institute patient navigation research program: methods, protocol, and measures. Cancer. 2008;113(12):3391–9.
5. Battaglia TA, Freund KM. Needs assessment of the breast health center at the women's health group. Boston: Boston Medical Center; 2001.
6. Freeman HP, Muth BJ, Kerner JF. Expanding access to cancer screening and clinical follow-up among the medically underserved. Cancer Pract. 1995;3(1):19–30.
7. Freeman HP. Patient navigation: a community centered approach to reducing cancer mortality. J Cancer Educ. 2006;21(1 Suppl):S11–4.
8. Freeman HP. Patient navigation: a community based strategy to reduce cancer disparities. J Urban Health. 2006;83(2):139–41.
9. Battaglia TA, Roloff K, Posner MA, Freund KM. Improving follow-up to abnormal breast cancer screening in an urban population. A patient navigation intervention. Cancer. 2007;109 (2 Suppl):359–67.
10. Bastani R, Yabroff KR, Myers RE, Glenn B. Interventions to improve follow-up of abnormal findings in cancer screening. Cancer. 2004;101(5 Suppl):1188–200.
11. Richards MA, Smith P, Ramirez AJ, Fentiman IS, Rubens RD. The influence on survival of delay in the presentation and treatment of symptomatic breast cancer. Br J Cancer. 1999; 79(5–6):858–64.
12. Richards MA, Westcombe AM, Love SB, Littlejohns P, Ramirez AJ. Influence of delay on survival in patients with breast cancer: a systematic review. Lancet. 1999;353(9159):1119–26.
13. Longest BB, Young GJ. Coordination and communitcation. In: Shortell SK, Kaluzny AD, eds. Health care management: organizational design and behavior, 4th edn. Albany, NY: Delmar Publishers; 2000. p. 237–275.
14. Phillips CE, Rothstein JD, Beaver K, Sherman BJ, Freund KM, Battaglia TA. Patient navigation to increase mammography screening among inner city women. J Gen Intern Med. 2010;26(2):123–9.
15. Battaglia TA, Bak S, Heeren T, et al. Boston patient navigation research program: the impact of navigation on time to diagnostic resolution after abnormal cancer screening. CEBP. 2012 In Press.
16. Mandyam V, McKinney R, Sherman BJ, Freund KM. Patient navigator assistance with screening mammography in an urban resident primary care practice. Oral Presentation at Society for General Internal Medicine Annual Meeting 2011, Pheonix AZ.
17. Battaglia TA, Parker VA, McCoy ME, et al. The Boston medical center patient navigation toolkit. 1st ed. Boston: The Avon Foundation for Women; 2012.
18. Parker VA, Clark JA, Leyson J, et al. Patient navigation: development of a protocol for describing what navigators do. Health Serv Res. 2010;45(2):514–31.
19. Battaglia TA, Burhansstipanov L, Murrell SS, Dwyer AJ, Caron SE. Assessing the impact of patient navigation: prevention and early detection metrics. Cancer. 2011;117(15 Suppl): 3553–64.
20. Kronman AC, Freund KM, Schoettler CL, et al. Developing metrics to improve the quality of a patient navigator breast health program. J Ambul Care Manage JACM. 2012 In Press.
21. Jean-Pierre P, Fiscella K, Winters PC, Paskett E, Wells K, Battaglia T. Cross-cultural validation of a patient satisfaction with interpersonal relationship with navigator measure: a multi-site patient navigation research study. Psychooncology. 2011.

Chapter 7
Consensus Support for the Role of Patient Navigation in the Nation's Healthcare System

Chrissy Liu, Rebecca Mason, Anne M. Roubal, Elizabeth Ojo, Elizabeth A. Calhoun and Steven R. Patierno

Purpose of the Patient Navigation Consensus Paper

Patient Navigation was developed as an intervention to improve outcomes among medically underserved populations by addressing barriers to completing a health care goal [1]. As Patient Navigation underwent widespread implementation, both its definition and practice evolved to address diverse patient populations and needs, by various workforce members, in numerous settings. This chapter is intended to create a common understanding of Patient Navigation and the role it can play in the healthcare system. It is aimed mainly at supporting recommendations for healthcare policy changes (e.g., staffing) and also provides a framework for building broad support for support for Patient Navigators across the healthcare delivery system.

C. Liu (✉)
Point B, Seattle, WA, USA
e-mail: cliu@pointb.com

R. Mason · E.A. Calhoun
Center for Population Science and Discovery, University of Arizona, Tucson, AZ, USA
e-mail: rebeccamason@email.arizona.edu

E.A. Calhoun
e-mail: ecalhoun@email.arizona.edu

A.M. Roubal
Population Health Sciences, University of Wisconsin, Madison, WI, USA
e-mail: aroubal@match.wisc.edu

E. Ojo
University of Michigan, Ann Arbor, MI, USA
e-mail: eojo@umich.edu

S.R. Patierno
Department of Medicine, Duke Cancer Institute, Durham, NC, USA
e-mail: steven.patierno@duke.edu

E.A. Calhoun and A. Esparza (eds.), *Patient Navigation*,
DOI 10.1007/978-1-4939-6979-1_7

The History of Patient Navigation

All people, regardless of socioeconomic level, education, race, or diagnosed disease, experience significant difficulties utilizing our complex systems of health care, thus Patient Navigation has the potential to benefit all. However, these difficulties are exacerbated among individuals facing complex chronic diseases as well as among vulnerable populations, making Patient Navigation even more important for those who experience numerous and challenging barriers [2]. In fact, research has demonstrated that Patient Navigation is most effective, and in many cases only effective, when targeted to populations with the largest barriers to care.

Patient Navigation can also serve to overcome barriers to health care and poor health outcomes that are exemplified among medically underserved populations. The Institute of Medicine issued a report entitled *Unequal Treatment: Confronting Racial and Ethnic Disparities in Health Care*, calling attention to disparities in quality care and access for racial and ethnic minorities and the uninsured [3]. The National Cancer Institute (NCI) defines "cancer health disparities" as "adverse differences in cancer incidence (new cases), cancer prevalence (all existing cases), cancer death (mortality), cancer survivorship, and burden of cancer or related health conditions that exist among specific population groups," [4] which may be characterized by age, disability, education, ethnicity, gender, geographic location, income, or race.

To address such health disparities, Dr. Harold Freeman created the first Patient Navigation program in 1990 in Harlem, New York. Navigators were recruited from the local community and trained to help to get women into the health system early to eliminate barriers between the point of suspicious finding and diagnostic resolution and treatment [1]. The results of the program in Harlem were remarkable. Before Patient Navigation was introduced in Harlem, in a 22-year period ending in 1986, 708 patients (94% black) with breast cancer were treated at Harlem Hospital Center. All of these patients were low income and half were uninsured. Women were offered free and low-cost examinations/mammograms as well as Patient Navigation services to remove barriers to ensure timely diagnostic resolution and the start of treatment. During the project from 1990 to 1992, 1034 females and 102 males were screened, of whom 7 breast cancers and 1 cervical cancer were found and 87.5% of those navigated with suspicious findings completed the breast biopsy process and only 56.6% of non-navigated group [1]. After the Patient Navigation intervention, the results were dramatically different in a positive way for the Harlem patients. Of 325 breast cancer patients, 41% of the patients had early stage breast cancer (0 and 1), 21% of the patients had stage 3 and 4; and the 5-year survival rate was 70% compared to 54 and 56% for stage 1 and 2, respectively, before program implementation [1].

The federal government took notice of the marked improvement with the work of Patient Navigators in Harlem and passed the Patient Navigation and Chronic Disease Prevention Act (H.R. 1812) ("Patient Navigation Act"), which was signed into law by President Bush in 2005 [5]. This landmark legislation helped to put a national reach to Patient Navigation by authorizing grant programs and by outlining six required responsibilities of nonmedical navigators including:

- Acting as liaisons by assisting in the coordination of healthcare services and provider referrals.
- Facilitating the involvement of community organizations in assisting individuals who are at risk for or who have cancer or other chronic diseases to receive better access to high-quality healthcare services.
- Notifying individuals of clinical trials and, on request, facilitating enrollment of eligible individuals in these trials.
- Anticipating, identifying, and helping patients to overcome barriers within the healthcare system.
- Coordinating with the relevant health insurance programs to provide information to individuals without health coverage.
- Conducting ongoing outreach to health disparity populations.

The goal of this effort was to design, implement, and evaluate replicable Patient Navigation programs targeting valuable populations. The Act defined Patient Navigation as "support and guidance offered to vulnerable populations with abnormal cancer screening or a cancer diagnosis with the goal of overcoming barriers to timely, quality care [6]." This Act authorized appropriations beginning in fiscal year 2006 and extending through the end of fiscal year 2010 [7]. Following this, in 2008, a U.S. Surgeons General collective issued a *National Call to Action on Cancer Prevention and Survivorship* and listed Patient Navigation one of the four priority areas the nation must embrace to make progress in the War on Cancer [8]. Lastly, with the passage of the Patient Protection and Affordable Care Act of 2010, the funding authorization for the Patient Navigation Act was extended through fiscal year 2015 as deemed necessary [9]. The Affordable Care Act (ACA) was a major step for Patient Navigation, reauthorizing Section 340a of the Public Health Service Act (Patient Navigator and Chronic Disease Prevention Act). The ACA mandates that insurance navigators help consumers navigate the health insurance marketplace. In addition, the ACA adds a requirement to ensure that all Patient Navigators meet minimum core proficiencies, to be defined by the Secretary of HHS [9].

Patient Navigation is explicitly mentioned in only one section of the ACA; however, the principles upon which the foundations of Patient Navigation are built can be seen throughout the act. The ACA provisions address four key issues imperative in reducing health disparities, all of which are amenable to increased implementation of Patient Navigation: prevention and early detection; healthcare access and coordination; insurance coverage and continuity; and diversity and cultural competency [10]. In 2012, the American College of Surgeons Commission on Cancer mandated that Patient Navigation is a standard of care that must be met by cancer programs seeking accreditation beginning in 2015 [11]. This requirement has led to a sharp increase in the number of cancer navigation programs in the country and, consequently, should increase the population of patients who will benefit from the proven ameliorative powers of Patient Navigation.

Research and Interest in Patient Navigation

In addition to the Harlem Hospital program, there have been other programs that have had demonstrable success with implementing Patient Navigation such as the Lincoln Medical and Mental Health Center, which saw a reduction in their colorectal cancer patient "no shows" from 67 to 10%, a decrease in time from initial appointment to treatment from 10 weeks to two weeks, and an increase in early detection by 50% [12]. This particular example also suggests that Patient Navigation holds potential for improving healthcare system efficiency and reducing costs (mitigating the negative time management and financial challenges associated with "no show" rates). Other successful Patient Navigation programs around the country are helping patients overcome financial, communication and systematic barriers [12]. "Overall, Patient Navigation programs are bringing about increases in screening, and adherence to diagnostic follow-up care after the detection of an abnormality [12]."

The National Cancer Institute Center to Reduce Health Disparities (NCI/CHCRD), the Health Resources and Services Administration (HRSA), the Centers for Medicare and Medicaid Services (CMS), the American Cancer Society (ACS), additional cancer advocacy organizations and even the pharmaceutical industry have all invested significant resources to fund Patient Navigation research and service delivery programs. This type of support has led to the growth of the field, and with continued support, the role of the navigator can become solidified as a permanent fixture in the health care professional space. As one example and as a result of the 2005 Patient Navigation Act, the NCI received $20 million to launch the Patient Navigation Research Program (PNRP) [13]. With additional support by the ACS, nine trial sites around the country were competitively selected to test the efficacy of a Patient Navigation intervention, specifically whether Patient Navigation decreases the delay between suspicious findings on screening to diagnostic resolution, and from diagnosis to the beginning of treatment. Analysis of research data from the nine sites demonstrated enhanced quality of life for cancer patients, greater satisfaction with the healthcare system, and increased rates of treatment commencement among other findings supporting the efficacy of Patient Navigation. More than 25 peer-reviewed papers have been published since this multi-center national trial was initiated: the majority of reports show consistent positive effects of Patient Navigation on minimizing diagnostic and treatment delays and maximizing diagnostic resolution.

In October 2008, the Health Resources and Services Administration awarded $4.8 million in total funding for six two-year projects with the intent to further investigate how Patient Navigators could improve health outcomes of patients battling chronic diseases [14]. HRSA awarded an additional ten Patient Navigation demonstration projects grants totaling $7.8 million in 2010. The Patient Navigator Outreach and Chronic Disease Prevention Program (PNDP) grantees provided navigation services to 11,574 patients mainly recruited in clinical settings through the work of 104 navigators and reached over 26,000 people through community outreach efforts such as health fairs, presentations, and educational sessions within various community settings that provided screenings and education about cancer and chronic diseases [14]. Navigators reported 52% of encounters involved coordinating healthcare services including scheduling and connecting patients to providers. Proactive navigation was also very common and a reported 45% of encounters dealt with follow-up and educating patients to ensure understanding of next steps in necessary health care [14]. Prior to the implementation of this program, at one site only 76% of patients clinic-wide kept scheduled appointments and patients who received navigation services increased to 100% attendance of scheduled medical appointments. By working to improve patients' health literacy and coordinating logistical aspects of care, navigators successfully delivered patient-centered care, proving Patient Navigator programs improve access, continuity, and effectiveness of care [14].

CMS already has a handful of community-based Patient Navigation programs through their Health Care Innovation Challenge Awards aimed at delivering better health, improved care, increased patient engagement, and lower healthcare costs [15]. Funded programs include the $15 million grant for a cancer-specific Patient Navigation program, Patient Care Connect Program (PCCP), through the University of Alabama at Birmingham's Comprehensive Cancer Center. The results of the study indicate a dramatic trend toward a clinically significant reduction in healthcare utilization and Medicare costs, with substantial impact during initial phase, survivorship and the last six months of life [16]. Specific results during the PCCP implementation include a drop in hospitalization rates of 19.7% and ICU admission rates were dramatically reduced by 6% compared to 0.8% in the non-navigated group [16]. In terms of Medicare claims, there was a considerable reduction of overall cost in the navigated patient population from $15,091 to $8269 per patient per quarter, which is a Medicare savings of $6822 per navigated patient; cost in the last six months of life decreased from $23,735 to $16,764 per patient for the navigated patient population, in comparison to the non-navigated group that increased from $13,418 to $15,544 [16]. CMS also funded a four-year $5.4 million national Cancer Prevention and Treatment Demonstration Project to determine if Patient Navigation can reduce cost and mortality of Medicare beneficiaries by decreasing barriers to cancer screening, promoting early detection and timely diagnosis, and enhancing access to treatment of cancer to the clinical core of the University of Texas, M.D. Anderson Cancer Center [17]. Project Facilitated Assistance, Research, and Outreach Services (FAROS) targets older Latino Medicare beneficiaries where participants are enrolled and randomized into either the intervention group of facilitated screening or treatment services by a trained Patient Navigator, or the comparison group of usual cancer prevention or treatment care [17]. As of 2010, over 1100 patients have enrolled in Project FAROS and of 821 baseline surveys, 36% of the navigated group reported never having a colorectal cancer screening (CRCS) [18]. The findings from Project FAROS will provide a tailored Patient Navigation intervention, inform public policy makers to decrease barriers to CRCS specific to older Latinos, as well as examine the economic impacts of Patient Navigation services.

There continues to be national interest in research around the field of Patient Navigation. The Patient-Centered Outcomes Research Institute (PCORI), an independent organization authorized by Congress as a result of the ACA, has funded research on health disparities and funds projects that utilize Patient Navigation. This nonprofit, nongovernmental entity is established to promote comparative effectiveness research by identifying research priorities, establishing a research agenda, and providing funding to conduct research that targets outcome differences in racial ethnic, and sex subpopulations [19]. In 2012, PCORI established addressing health disparities as a research priority. In releasing its funding guidelines, it stated that one example of a fundable research project that intends to answer "How does the availability of a Patient Navigator for patients and/or caregivers improve patients' health outcomes compared to usual strategies? Under what circumstances, or for what conditions, are Patient Navigators most effective [20]?" Currently, almost half of the projects funded by PCORI's Addressing Disparities program include interventions containing a CHW-Patient Navigator component, and almost all of those projects target racial and ethnic minority groups [20]. There is already evidence to support Patient Navigation as a method to improve outcomes related to the screening and diagnosis of cancer [1, 6, 10, 12, 13, 16, 17].

Recognizing the value in the services of Patient Navigators, the American College of Surgeon's Commission on Cancer (COC) and the Association of Community Cancer Centers have both placed an emphasis on the creation of Patient Navigation services [11, 21]. The COC guidelines actually require accredited cancer treatment facilities to have a Patient Navigation program by January 2015 or risk losing that status. There are currently over 1500 COC accredited facilities responsible for treating approximately 70% of the newly diagnosed cancer cases [22].

Moving Patient Navigation Forward

Patient Navigation has evolved over the years. It is being used in other chronic disease fields and now covers the entire cancer continuum from outreach (screening navigation) through diagnosis into treatment and through survivorship or end of life. Originating as trained lay community health workers helping patients overcome access to care barriers, the Patient Navigation field has grown into positions for health care professionals, including nurses and social workers, as well as highly trained outreach workers that help coordinate care for patients and to serve on a multidisciplinary team [23]. In fact, the Oncology Nursing Society, the Association of Oncology Social Work, and the National Association of Social Work have issued a joint position statement about Patient Navigation and its role as an essential component of cancer care services [24]. They agree that the navigation processes are "fundamental in nursing and social work" and that they both "enhance their professional knowledge and competencies with preparation in Patient Navigation processes [24].” Additionally, there is support for including lay navigators (defined as a trained nonprofessional) with nursing and social work navigators as part of a multidisciplinary team. Patient Navigators, both professional and lay, enhance the healthcare team, as their primary role is to help the patient through the labyrinthine healthcare system and reduce or eliminate barriers to care. Some of the most common barriers patients face are geographic access to the clinic or hospital, identification and access to financial services, transportation and child care issues, fear and anxiety, medical mistrust, lost wages and language and cultural issues [23] (Fig. 7.1).

The evolution of Patient Navigation over the past 20 years has allowed for diverse patient needs to be addressed by varied workforce members across several diseases and settings and has led to improved outcomes for patients, which is also a benefit to the healthcare system. Notwithstanding, the presence of Patient Navigation is fragmented in the healthcare system and its contribution is consistently misunderstood. One example of this is in the discussion around the requirements for establishing the state health insurance exchanges under the ACA. The Department of Health and Human Services has set the requirement that states creating a state run exchange “must establish or have a process in place to establish and operate a Navigator program [25].” Most recently, in September 2015 CMS awarded $67 million in Navigator Cooperative Agreement Awards to individuals and organizations to serve as navigators in federally facilitated partnership exchanges/marketplaces [26]. The goals of the program are to support the staffing of navigators who serve as insurance eligibility and enrollment specialists; provide information in a fair and impartial manner; facilitate the selection of a qualified health plan; provide referrals to the health insurance consumer assistance or state ombudsman; and provide culturally and linguistically appropriate information [27]. With the federal government’s continued support of cancer and chronic disease

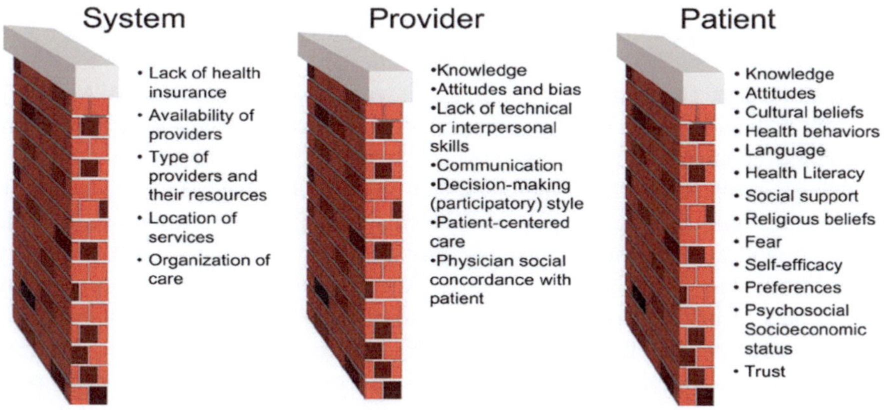

Fig. 7.1 Common barriers to care. Reprinted from Seminars in Nephrology, Vol. 33(5), Nicholas SB, Kalantar-Zadeh K, Norris KC. Racial disparities in kidney disease outcomes, Pages 409–15, Copyright 2013, with permission from Elsevier

Patient Navigation programs, it is uncertain why, in the creation of the state exchange guidelines, the term navigator was used for an insurance enrollment specialist. This inconsistent use of the term highlights the need for a clearly defined role of Patient Navigators.

Recommendation #1: Establish a Job Description and Recognized Job Code for Patient Navigators

Patient Navigation was established in 1990 and despite the growth of the field and several federally funded programs, the Department of Labor Standard Occupational Classification does not recognize the job title of 'Patient Navigator'. This classification is used by Federal statistical agencies to classify workers into occupational categories for the purpose of collecting, calculating, or disseminating data [28]. One of the key challenges in Patient Navigation is the need to clearly define terms and roles to distinguish it from other health professions. Patient Navigation can be described as an intervention that assists individuals in overcoming barriers to timely access to the full continuum of quality healthcare. Although all individuals would benefit from Patient Navigation, it is a particularly effective intervention to reduce health disparities in cancer care when aimed at vulnerable or medically underserved populations and functions as a system [29]. Patient Navigation can include not only patients but also providers, families, and caregivers, and extend throughout the cancer continuum from prevention and screening through post-treatment and survivorship.

Given that the Patient Navigator role was born from using women in the community to help steer their peers into screening and care along the continuum, there still seems to be some confusion between the role of a Patient Navigator and a community health worker (CHW). While the term 'Community Health Worker' is often an umbrella phrase that includes among other roles, Patient Navigation, it was recently recognized with a Standard Occupational Classification after a recommendation by the Department of Labor, and it was also included in the ACA [9, 30]. A CHW is defined as one that "assists individuals and communities to adopt healthy behaviors, conducts outreach for medical personnel or health organizations to implement programs in the community that promote, maintain, and improve individual and community health, provides information on available resources, provide social support and informal counseling, advocates for individuals and community health needs, provides services such as first aid and blood pressure screening, may collect data to help identify community health needs" [30]. Thus, at present it is widely recognized that the roles of Patient Navigators and CHWs are not identical, but are synergistic and complementary. To use a common metaphor, CHWs raise health awareness and focus more on moving people "to the front door" of needed health care, whereas Patient Navigators help people get "through the door" and through the labyrinthine healthcare system behind the door (Fig. 7.2). Patient

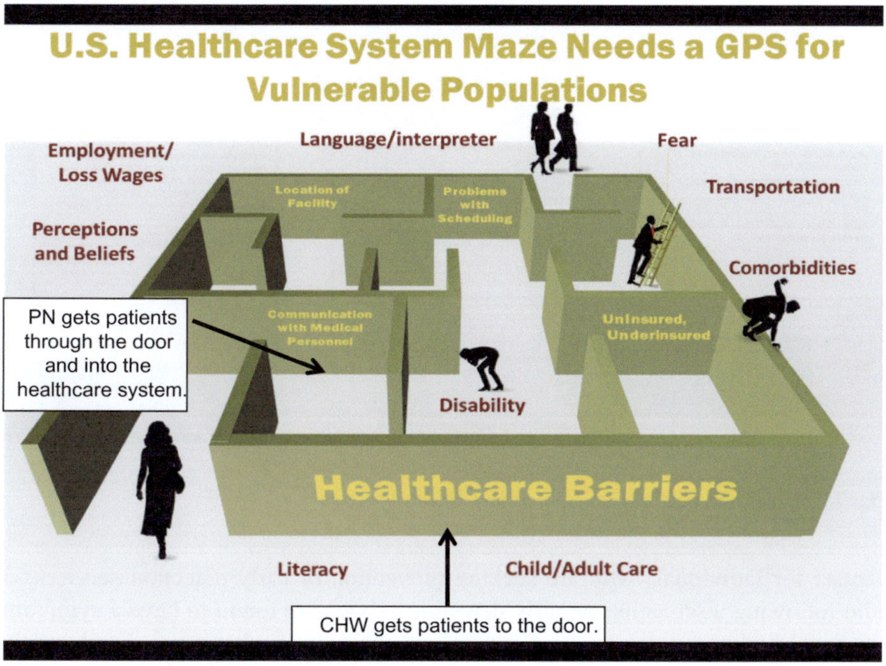

Fig. 7.2 The role of delineation between Patient Navigators and Community Health Workers. Reprinted from U.S. Department of Health and Human Services. Patient Navigation Research Program (PNRP). March 8, 2010. 45th Regular Meeting of the Board of Scientific Advisors Center to Reduce Cancer Health Disparities. U.S. Healthcare System Maze Needs a GPS for Vulnerable Populations. Available from: http://deainfo.nci.nih.gov/advisory/bsa/archive/bsa0310/presentations/915%20Chu%20Paskett%20Howerton%20%20BSA%20PNRP%20Presentation_3%205%2010_FINAL.pdf

Navigation is focused on helping people overcome barriers to health care, whether the barriers are structural (such as lack of insurance or transportation) or psychosocial (such as fear or medical mistrust).

While this lack of clarity in the healthcare system is not an uncommon occurrence because of some overlap in these roles, there are distinct differences that need to be made in order to move the field of Patient Navigation forward (Fig. 7.3). CHWs promote positive health behaviors in the community, use evidence-based interventions to educate community members, encourage appropriate health screenings, and can help people enroll in health insurance programs, among other tasks [31, 32]. The ACA of 2010 supports this definition of the role of the CHW as it provided grant opportunities from the CDC over 4 years to enhance programming efforts across the nation [31].

The role of Patient Navigation is different but complementary, as further delineated in another section of health reform legislation, supporting for Patient Navigation programs through HRSA demonstration projects [14]. There the role of Patient Navigation is explicit and in affirming that Navigators must: 1. Serve as a

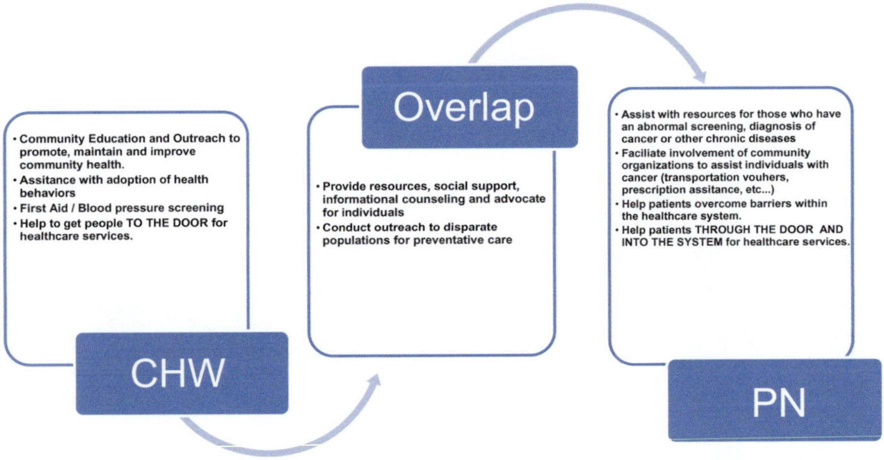

Fig. 7.3 Patient Navigation and Community Health Workers

contact for individuals who are seeking prevention or early detection services, or who following a screening or early detection service are found to have a symptom, abnormal finding, or diagnosis of cancer, or other chronic disease; 2. Facilitate the involvement of community organizations in assisting individuals who are at risk for cancer or other chronic diseases to receive better access to high-quality health services; 3. Notify individuals of clinical trials, and on request, facilitate enrollment of eligible individuals in these trials; 4. Anticipate, identify, and help patients to overcome barriers within the healthcare system to ensure prompt diagnostic resolution of an abnormal finding or cancer or other chronic disease; 5. Coordinate with the relevant health insurance ombudsman programs to provide information to individuals who are at risk for or who have cancer or other chronic diseases about health coverage, including private insurance, health care savings accounts, and other publically funded programs; and 6. Conduct ongoing outreach to health disparity populations, including the uninsured, rural populations, and other medically underserved populations, in addition to assisting other individuals who are at risk for or who have cancer or other chronic diseases to seek preventative care [33]. Implicit in this description of Patient Navigator functions compared to CHW's is that most Patient Navigators are employed by the health systems that they function within, whereas most CHWs are employed by municipal, county, or state agencies. It bears repeating: CHW's focus on getting people "to" the front door of a health system, whereas Patient Navigators focus on getting them "through" the complex healthcare delivery system.

The health care system continues to struggle with how to address health disparities, including access to care, quality of care, and high healthcare costs. Patient Navigation is one way to systematically address the fragmented healthcare system. However, although there are several highly effective training programs spread across the country, there are currently no standardized professional trainings with a defined minimum core curriculum. Given that these positions often rely on grant funding, there can be high turnover and low job security. Since Patient Navigation services are not recognized as reimbursable, there is often little incentive to create a sustainable role in the community or healthcare institution they serve.

Recommendation #2: Create National Standards for Training and Certification of Patient Navigation

Currently there is an array of Patient Navigation programs across the country; however, there is also a lack of national standards for training. The existing navigation training programs include a range of interactive classroom instruction while others are online or use a mixed-method approach. The length can range from 160 classroom hours to six weeks to three days of instruction. These training programs vary in length, target audience, attendee requirement/pre-requisite, content focus, and mode of delivery. Along with these differences, Patient Navigators vary with educational and healthcare experience and it is imperative to establish an adequate preparation regardless of job title, patient population, disease condition, or practice setting that enables Patient Navigators to teach patients the individualized steps to take for successful navigation in the health system; patients can then gain the skills to take ownership of their health. This diversity has implications for the intricacy of curricula materials and methods of delivery for an accepted, definitive training program.

Although there is a lack of agreement on development and maintenance of effective Patient Navigator training programs, the dissemination of core competencies of training topics necessary to excel as a Patient Navigator can be derived from the NCI's PNRP, CMS, and ACS standardized programs [23]. All three programs employ Patient Navigators who are trained, culturally competent healthcare workers who help patients to subjugate barriers to access quality care and negotiate through the health system. Cumulatively, the programs developed the standardized curriculum of training topics based upon core competencies from current navigators and training experts at the nine PNRP sites, the NCI and the ACS in July 2006 [23]. These include an overview of health and cancer disparities and thus the inception of Patient Navigation; the varying roles, responsibilities, and programs for Patient Navigation; cancer overview with a focus on screening and treatment; culture and diversity; effective communication and client interaction skills; introduction to clinical research; health system mapping and community assessment; and resource management [23]. The training was delivered using interactive formats to target different learning styles through the use of traditional lecture, small group discussion, and roleplay with case scenarios.

Following this precedence, The Harold P. Freeman Patient Navigation Institute (HPFPNI) was established in 2007 to support the growth in Patient Navigation programs by offering standards and best practices of navigator training that are customizable for each program. The Institute, located in New York City, serves as a gold standard of Patient Navigation and offers a certification upon completion of the two-day in-person training, which ensures programs uphold best practices and adhere to the peer-reviewed, recognized definition of Patient Navigation set forth by PNRP [34]. HPFPNI has trained over a thousand people the skills of successful Patient Navigators through the core principles such as informing the timely necessity of certain examinations, eliminating barriers to timely care across the healthcare continuum, and the critical function of overcoming barriers to timely diagnosis and treatment in patients with abnormal findings [34].

A training program that focuses on competencies enables individuals to be well prepared to perform their job duties in a real-world setting. Further, competency-based approaches facilitate multidisciplinary teams and programs that effectively work together to address the complexity of cross-cutting problems that are often experienced in a setting such as health care (Chapter 20). The previously described standardized Patient Navigator training program (ACS, CMS, NCI-PNRP) utilized the core competencies as a guide to develop a performance checklist, taking the first step toward an accepted definition of core competencies for navigators [23]. This checklist was adapted from Denver Health's CHW Competency Assessment Tool, which was designed to test proficiency as a CHW though skills-testing prior to graduating the program and earning the certificate [35]. The core curriculum for this CHW training program is performance based and addresses three areas of emphasis: workplace/academic core, vocational core, and cooperative education core/CHW field experience. The assessment tool contains elements of competencies and application of skills and knowledge presented during the training in real-world situations like basic interviewing skills, familiarizing the client with the agency, basic health needs assessment, health promotion and education, resource referral, and follow-up [35]. From the CHW assessment tool, the four broad areas adapted for the Patient Navigator checklist include client interaction; care management (health assessment and advising); intervention (referrals); and documentation [23]. The tool is given at the beginning of the CHW program and used as a reference throughout the training to develop and support effective competencies.

Established competencies for similar fields to Patient Navigation are currently the foundation for accreditation or certification at either state or national levels (Chapter 20). As of October 2014, Illinois House bill 5412 defines CHW's core competencies and roles and focuses on developing a certification process; in Texas and Indiana, the state health departments are the accrediting body for the CHW training programs [31]. Texas, Ohio, and Minnesota require a certification of CHWs to cover services. Additionally in Indiana and Alaska, only programs that provide standardized CHW training are allowed to pay for CHW professionals. However, the New Mexico Senate bill 58 allows for voluntary CHW certification [31]. Minnesota and Massachusetts have both taken comprehensive approaches to implement systems of policy change to build capacity for an integrated and sustainable CHW workforce; Patient Navigation can use CHWs as a model to determine the necessity of credentialing or State certification [31].

By ensuring the stewardship of scare resources, training in core competencies (Chapter xx), and acquisition of basic skills and knowledge [23], a national training and certification program using established national standards can propel the field of Patient Navigation to the next level by establishing and securing the importance of this role in the health care system.

Recommendation #3: Demonstrate the Usefulness of Patient Navigation on Improving Healthcare Quality

The ACA called for a national strategy to improve the delivery of healthcare services, patient health outcomes and population health [9]. The National Strategy for Quality Improvement in Health Care (the National Quality Strategy) established three aims and six priorities for quality improvement [36]. The aims of the Strategy are to (1) improve the overall quality of care by making care more patient-centered, reliable, accessible, and safe; (2) improve the health of the US population by supporting proven interventions to address behavioral, social, and environmental determinants of health; and (3) reduce the cost of quality healthcare [36]. To advance the aims, six priorities were set through a participatory process of national stakeholders: (1) making care safer by reducing harm caused in the delivery of care; (2) ensuring that each person and family are engaged as partners in their care; (3) promoting effective communication and coordination of care; (4) promoting the most effective prevention and treatment practices for the leading causes of mortality, starting with cardiovascular disease; (5) working with communities to promote wide use of best practices to enable healthy living; and (6) making quality care more affordable for individuals, families, employers, and governments by developing and spreading new health care delivery models [36] (Fig. 7.4). Five out of six of these priorities clearly align with the goals of Patient Navigation with synergistic efforts of CHWs, as outlined in priority five, to work within communities to enable healthy living and assist people to needed and available health care.

In the 2012 Annual Report to Congress, the National Quality Strategy provided long-term goals for each of its established priorities. One of these goals for engaging patients and families is to enable patients and their families and caregivers to navigate, coordinate, and manage their care appropriately and effectively [36]. Two of the long-term goals for promoting effective communication and coordination of care include: improving the quality of care transitions and communications across care settings and establishing shared accountability and integration of communities and healthcare systems to improve quality care and reduce health disparities [36]. Clearly, the role of a Patient Navigator can help achieve these important goals.

In terms of the priority for promoting the best prevention and treatment practices for the leading cause of mortality, the strategy is choosing to first focus on cardiovascular disease; it may be beneficial for Patient Navigators to play a role in achieving the goals for this chronic disease. Following a cardiac event or procedure,

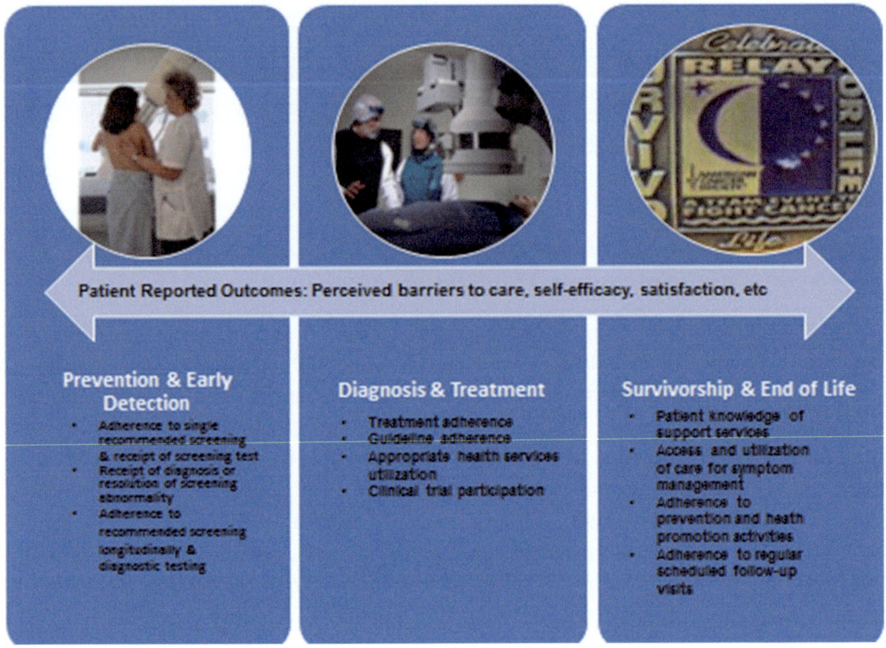

Fig. 7.4 Roles of Patient Navigators

awareness of and enrollment in outpatient cardiac rehabilitation (OCR) remains suboptimal and the use of a Patient Navigation is a proven practice and intervention to improve these outcomes. Minority women receive 12% fewer referrals than white women for OCR following hospital discharge for a cardiac event, illustrating a major health disparity that can be eliminated through Patient Navigation [37]. Compared to usual care, participants receiving navigation were six times more likely to have an awareness of OCR and of those patients proved nine times more likely to enroll in OCR following hospital discharge [38].

Lastly, with the priority of making quality care more affordable, the goal is to ensure affordable and accessible quality healthcare for all. Clearly it is important to look into payment reforms and establishing common measures to assess the costs impacts of new programs and payment systems. There is an opportunity here to build on the work of the PNRP and CMS programs, which have begun to address the question of cost-effectiveness of Patient Navigation, as well as the success of the CHW model as guidance in moving this goal forward.

In addition to coalition building among service providers, local and state governments, professionals and the community, CHWs have made significant advancements in several states by integrating their work into the healthcare system through the use of empirical evidence. In Minnesota, the Community Health Worker Alliance successfully lobbied the state legislature by demonstrating the Return on Investment (ROI) of paying for training and education of CHW's relative to the benefit to the community [39]. In Massachusetts, CHWs helped more than 200,000 uninsured people enroll in health insurance programs, when the state health law reform took effect [39]. A study of CHWs found that they increased access to primary care through culturally competent outreach and enrollment and improved quality and cost-effectiveness of care by assisting patients with self-management of chronic diseases [40]. However, the financing of these workers can be diverse. In Alaska, CHWs are funded by the corporations that employ them. In Massachusetts, funding comes from the state budget; while in Minnesota and Indiana, the work of the CHW is reimbursable under the state Medicaid programs [39]. Patient Navigation programs can learn from these models of engaging stakeholders, developing national standards for training programs and accreditation in order to enhance their role on a multidisciplinary team and solidify their presence in the healthcare delivery system.

With a national priority on quality improvement in healthcare, Patient Navigation is poised to promote a more patient-centric health care service delivery model, integrate a fragmented health care system for the benefit of the patients, and eliminate barriers to timely and appropriate care and thus reduce the cost of quality care. As we move to value-based care, the payment mechanisms will allow for Patient Navigators to be part of the team in the bundled payment models.

Recommendation #4: Support Research in Patient Navigation

With the current national focus on patient-centered care, it is important to consider developing additional research and validated patient-reported outcome metrics since patients have stated that Patient Navigators are effective because they provide emotional support, as well as information and assistance with problem-solving. Now there is an opportunity to evaluate the impact of Patient Navigation in improving cancer outcomes beyond the detection and diagnosis phase of care.

The National Cancer Institute (NCI) Community Cancer Centers Program is a network of hospital cancer centers that serves as a community-based platform to support basic, clinical, and population-based research initiatives across the cancer care continuum—from prevention, screening, diagnosis, treatment, and survivorship through end-of-life care [41]. In 2007, the NCI provided funding to 16 community cancer centers at hospitals around the country for a pilot program called the NCI Community Cancer Centers Program (NCCCP). The pilot was designed to build a community-based research platform to support a wide range of basic, clinical, and population-based research on cancer prevention, screening, diagnosis, treatment, survivorship, and palliative care at community hospitals—contributing to enhanced quality of care for patients and advancing cancer research. On August 12, 2009, the NCCCP received funding through the NIH Evaluation Office to conduct a comparative analysis of NCCCP sites with comparable community cancer centers external to the NCCCP [42]. Increased quality of care among NCCCP sites was significantly greater than that among comparison-group hospitals for radiation therapy after breast-conserving surgery and hormonal therapy for women with hormone receptor-positive breast cancer. In multivariate regressions, increases in hormonal therapy among NCCCP-site patients were significantly greater than those among comparison-group hospitals [43]. As a result of funding from the American Recovery and Reinvestment Act (ARRA) in 2010, the NCCCP expanded the original pilot network from 16 to 30 hospitals in 22 states. A new evaluation is planned for the 14 additional sites [43]. This analysis will build on the ongoing evaluation by understanding how the NCCCP has enhanced cancer care delivery to patients. NCCCP cancer centers promote multidisciplinary cancer care that is patient-centered, data-driven, evidence-based, and delivered through coordinated teams of physicians, Patient Navigators, and staff in a community setting.

Although Patient Navigation has mostly been used in oncology, it does not need to be limited to cancer. In response to CMS's quality improvements initiatives (QI) such as imposed financial penalties to hospitals with high 30-day readmission rates, PCORI awarded $2 million for their project PArTNER, Patient Navigator to Reduce Readmissions, to African American and minority-serving institutions, who provide care for patients with limited social support, health literacy and contribute most to readmission rates [44]. Tailoring to the needs of the patients they serve, navigators personally visit during hospitalization and at home post-discharge to provide social support and self-management skills training, followed by ongoing patient/caregiver-led telephone support, which timely has great potential to impact QI [44]. In 2014, PCORI awarded over $1.8 million to address chronic hepatitis B virus (HBV) infection (CHB) rates in Asian Americans, the highest in the US and the largest health gap compared to white Americans. Using Patient Navigators plus mobile phone text messaging intervention compared to usual care, this study hopes to improve timely testing every 6–12 months for patients at high risk for complications and early signs of liver problems [45].

Recommendation #5: Explore Reimbursement Models for Patient Navigation

Given the growth of the field of Patient Navigation and its potential impact on the health system for not only cancer, but other chronic diseases as well, it is important to explore reimbursement models for the services provided by Patient Navigators. The goal for Patient Navigation would be permanent integration into the healthcare delivery system and recognition as a covered service for both public and private payers. There are two important models to consider as guidance for pursing reimbursement models: diabetes educators and CHWs.

In 1997, the federal government made some important changes to Medicare in the Balanced Budget Act of 1997. Not only was coverage for some clinical cancer screening services expanded, but it also extended coverage to include diabetes self-management [46]. This expansion covered diabetes self-management education and training when provided to an individual with diabetes by a certified provider in an outpatient setting [46]. Physicians providing care to the patient must certify that the services are needed under a comprehensive plan of care to ensure therapy compliance or to provide the patient with diabetes self-management skills and knowledge [46]. The training must be completed by a "certified provider" defined by Medicare as "a physician, other individual or entity paid under Medicare's physician fee schedules who meets the National Diabetes Advisory Board (NDAB) standards [47]." Medicare must actually receive a copy of the certified provider's Education Recognition Program (ERP) certificate from the American Diabetes Associate (ADA) before any claims can be submitted for this service.

Given the evolution of the research, standardized training and the impact on patient outcomes, diabetes education, and training is now a reimbursable expense for both public and private payors. As of mid-2016, 46 states and the District of Columbia have some law that requires health insurance policy coverage for diabetes treatment. Laws in Mississippi and Missouri require only that insurers offer coverage, but not necessarily include the coverage in all active policies. Most states require coverage for both direct treatment and for diabetes equipment and supplies that are often used by the patient at home [48]. Both private insurance and public insurance offer billing codes for the services of the diabetes educator in increments of 30–60 min [47].

Congress also created the CMS Innovation Center under the ACA, giving the Center the authority and direction to "test innovative payment and service delivery models to reduce program expenditures, while preserving or enhancing the quality of care" for those who get Medicare, Medicaid, or CHIP benefits [9]. The Center's mandate gives it great flexibility in selecting and testing innovative payment and service delivery models, enables the Center to work with Medicare, State Medicaid, and CHIP programs to better serve beneficiaries, and provides $10 billion in direct funding in fiscal years 2011 through 2019 to support this mission. It also allows the Secretary of Health and Human Services to expand, through rulemaking, the scope and duration of models proven effective after evaluation, including implementation on a nationwide basis to cover the entire Medicare, Medicaid, or CHIP populations.

In September 2012, H.R. 6521 was introduced at the federal level to "provide payment for Patient Navigator services under title XIX of the Social Security Act" [49]. The Bill, which called for reimbursement of "any Patient Navigator service" as specified by the Patient Navigation Act, provided to a Medicaid beneficiary, however, did not pass [49], as well as the more recently proposed Patient Navigation Assistance Act of 2014 that amended title XIX of the Social Security Act—otherwise known as Medicaid—to require that state Medicaid plans provide reimbursement for Patient Navigation services [17]. As Medicaid provides coverage to minority and low-income individuals this would be a particularly innovative way to target the population most in need of Patient Navigation services in the context of a complex, changing healthcare environment. Patient Navigators can not only facilitate improved healthcare access and quality for underserved populations through advocacy and care coordination, but they can also address deep-rooted issues related to distrust in providers and the health system that often lead to avoidance of health problems and non-compliance with treatment recommendations [50].

Similar to the evolution for the reimbursement of diabetes educators, CHWs are starting to follow suit with reimbursement efforts for the services. Leading the way is the state of Minnesota. However, before the state legislature took action, Minnesota committed to a statewide initiative whose mission was to reduce cultural and linguistic barriers to health care, improve quality and cost-effectiveness of care, and increase the number of healthcare workers who come from diverse backgrounds or underserved communities [51]. The project of the initiative developed a standardized curriculum to educate CHWs in Minnesota; developed professional standards for CHWs that define their role in the healthcare delivery system; created a sustainable employment market, incorporating CHW's into the healthcare workforce; and demonstrated that trained CHWs are effective, and that a CHW's time with a patient is a billable/reimbursable valued service [51]. As a result of advocacy efforts to the state legislature, the service of CHWs became eligible for reimbursement [52]. The work being done in Minnesota is also groundbreaking in that the state Medicaid program covers reimbursement for the work being done by CHWs. In order to qualify for reimbursement, the CHW must complete the state's fourteen-credit certificate program and at that point, are eligible to enroll in the Minnesota Health Care Plan as a Medicaid provider authorized to serve under supervision of approved billing providers [39].

Patient Navigation can also learn from both the diabetes educator and CHW paths towards reimbursement. In recent years, several states have bundled payments for CHWs as part of non-clinician members in care teams. The same can be extended to Patient Navigators depending on the care delivery model used and the risk appetite of the physicians and healthcare organizations. Patient-centered medical homes and ACA Section 2703 Health Homes are two popular care delivery models pursued by state Medicaid programs for reimbursing community health workers [9]. Under these models, physician practices and healthcare organizations develop care teams by recruiting new staff or training existing staff such as nurses and medical assistants for patient education, care coordination, and population health monitoring. The care teams are typically reimbursed on a per-member-per-month basis by Medicaid, Medicare, and state's commercial insurers. Health Homes established under Section 2703 of the ACA, which serve Medicaid beneficiaries with two or more chronic conditions or persistent mental health condition are also eligible to receive an enhanced federal match for the services delivered in the first 8 quarters of implementation [53]. As of March 2014, 47 states had implemented medical homes or health homes. Patient Navigation services can be delivered as part of these medical homes to help enrollees navigate the healthcare system. Other care delivery models in which CHWs and Patient Navigators can be incorporated and reimbursed include accountable care organizations (ACO) and shared community-based resources. Under shared resources programs, state Medicaid reimburses for resources shared by multiple practices and organizations to coordinate care. Size of these shared resource teams range from single care managers to large inter-disciplinary teams, and they are often reimbursed using a per-member-per-month rate. Accountable care organizations (ACO) are typically responsible for providing care across a variety of settings including primary care and acute care. Since ACOs need to provide culturally appropriate support to members for navigating the healthcare system, they typically include community health workers and potentially Patient Navigators. Payments for non-clinician members such as CHWs and Patient Navigators can be bundled into payment strategies for ACOs which includes one of the following [54]:

- One-Sided Shared Savings—Modified fee-for-service model in which care teams share a portion of the savings, but not the losses.
- Two-Sided Shared Savings—Modified fee-for-service model in which care teams share both benefits (portion of savings) and losses.
- Bundled payments—Care teams are reimbursed single payment for one episode of care for a patient, which might include multiple services.
- Partial capitation/global payments—Care teams receive partial capitation payment for certain services
- Global payments—Care teams receive fixed monthly or annual payment per patients (per-member-per-month) regardless of services provided.

Implications/Conclusion

The momentum in health care is to improve quality and access to care as well as empower patients to have a leading role in their care. Given the decades of experience and data collected in Patient Navigation programs, it is clear that this role is critical in addressing the healthcare disparities that plague our society.

With policy initiatives in job classification, certification and training, quality and research, Patient Navigation can continue to grow as an integral part of the healthcare delivery system. The ACA reauthorizes Section 340a of the PHSA, the Patient Navigator and Chronic Disease Prevention grants for five more years through 2015 [9]. There was an additional important requirement added to this revision, which states that in order for an entity to receive a grant, it must ensure the navigators meet minimum core proficiencies tailored to the specific intervention [9]. While authorization levels beyond fiscal year 2015 were not specified, it is imperative that the advocates integrate Patient Navigation into the fabric of the healthcare delivery system across the country.

References

1. Freeman HP, Muth BJ, Kerner JF. Expanding access to cancer screening and clinical follow-up among medically underserved. Cancer Pract. 1995;3(1):19–30.
2. Moy B, Chabner BA. Patient Navigator programs, cancer disparities, and the patient protection and affordable care act. Oncologist. 2011;16(7):926–9.
3. Institute of Medicine. Unequal treatment: confronting racial and ethnic disparities in health care. Washington, DC: National Academies Press; 2003. Available at www.nap.edu/openbook.php?record-_id=12875&page=R1.

4. National Cancer Institute. Available at http://crchd.cancer.gov/disparities/defined.html.
5. United States Government Printing Office. Patient Navigation Outreach and Chronic Disease Prevention Act. Public Law 109-18, 119 STAT. 340. Congress. 29 June 2005. Available at www.gpo.gov/fdsys/pkg/BILLS-109hr1812enr/pdf/BILLS-109hr1812enr.pdf/.
6. Hopkins J, Mumber MP. Patient Navigation through the cancer care continuum: an overview. J. Oncol. Pract. 2009;5(4):150.
7. Pub. L. 109–18, June 29, 2005, 119 Stat. 340 Short title, see 42 U.S.C. 201 note.
8. Cabe J, Springer S. National call to action on cancer prevention and survivorship. Tucson, AZ: Excel Print Communications; 2008.
9. United States Government Printing Office. Patient Protection and Affordable Care Act. Public Law 111-147, 124 Stat. 119, §3510. 23 March 2010. Available at http://www.gpo.gov/fdsys/pkg/PLAW-111publ148/pdf/PLAW-111publ148.pdf.
10. Natale-Pereira A, Enard KR, Nevarez L, Jones LA. The role of Patient Navigators in eliminating health disparities. Cancer. 2011;117(15 0):3543–52.
11. The American College of Surgeons, Commission on Cancer. Cancer program standards 2012: ensuring patient centered care. Available at http://www.facs.org/cancer/coc/cocprogramstandards2012.pdf.
12. Varner A, Murph P. Cancer Patient Navigation: where do we go from here? Oncol Issues. 2010;52.
13. Freund K, Battaglia T, Calhoun E, Dudley D, Fiscella K, Paskett E, Raich P, Roetzheim R, Patient Navigation Research Program Group. National cancer institute Patient Navigation research program: methods, protocol, and measures. Cancer. 2008;113(12):3391–9.
14. Department of Health and Human Services. Health Resources and Services Administration. Report to U.S. Congress. Patient Navigator Outreach and Chronic Disease Prevention Program. Available at http://www.hrsa.gov/about/organization/bureaus/bhw/reportstocongress/patientnavigatoroutreach.pdf.
15. Department of Health and Humans Services. Centers for Medicare & Medicaid Services. Health Care Innovation Award Profiles. Available at http://innovations.cms.gov/initiatives/innovation-awards/project-profiles.html.
16. Thannickal B. Preliminary UAB study shows dramatic trend of cost savings in lay navigation program for cancer patients. June 2015. Available at https://www.uab.edu/news/focus-on-patient-care/item/6122-preliminary-uab-study-shows-dramatic-trend-of-cost-savings-in-lay-navigation-program-for-cancer-patients.
17. King D, Miranda P, Gor B, et al. Addressing cancer health disparities using a global "biopsychosocial" approach Addressing global cancer health disparities. Cancer. 2010;116 (2):264–9.
18. National *Dialogue for Action* Poster Session presenters; 2009. Pg. 3. Available at http://preventcancer.org/wp-content/uploads/2015/12/poster-session2009.pdf.
19. Patient Centered Outcomes Research Institute. Available at http://www.pcori.org.
20. Patient Centered Outcomes Research Institute. Funding Announcement: Addressing Disparities. (May 22, 2012): 9. Available at http://www.pcori.org/assets/PFA-Addressing-Disparities-05222012.pdf.
21. The American Association of Community Cancer Centers Cancer Program Guidelines. 2009. Available at http://acc-cancer.org/publications/pdf/publications_cpguidelines.pdf.
22. The American College of Surgeons, Commission on Cancer. Available at http://www.facs.org/cancerprogram/.
23. Calhoun EA, Whitley EM, Esparza A, Ness E, Greene A, Garcia R, et al. A national Patient Navigator training program. Health Promot Pract. 2010;11:205–15.
24. Oncology Nursing Society, the Association of Oncology Social Work, and the National Association of Social Workers Joint Position on the Role of Oncology Nursing and Oncology Social Work in Patient Navigation. 2010. Available at http://www.aosw.org/docs/PR-PositionPatientNav.pdf.

25. Department of Health and Human Services. Centers for Medicare and Medicaid Services. Blueprint for Approval of Affordable State-based and State Partnership Insurance Exchanges. Available at http://www.cciio.cms.gov/resources/files/hie-blueprint-081312.pdf.
26. Department of Health and Human Services. Centers for Medicare and Medicaid Services. Cooperative Agreement to Support Navigators in Federally-facilitated and State Partnership Marketplaces. Initial Announcement 2015. Available at https://www.cms.gov/CCIIO/Programs-and-Initiatives/Health-Insurance-Marketplaces/Downloads/Navigator_2015_FOA_FINAL_04_15_2015.pdf.
27. 45 C.F.R. 115.210. Navigator Program Standards.
28. Department of Labor. Standard Occupational Classification. Available at http://www.bls.gov/soc/home.htm.
29. Vargas RB, Ryan GW, et al. Characteristics of the original Patient Navigation programs to reduce disparities in the diagnosis and treatment of breast cancer. Cancer. 2008;113(2):426.
30. Department of Labor. Bureau of Labor Statistics. Standard Occupational Classification (SOC)—21-1094 Community Health Workers. 2010. Available at http://www.bls.gov/soc/2010/soc211094.htm.
31. Centers for Disease Control National Center for Chronic Disease Prevention and Health Promotion, Division of Heart Disease and Stroke Prevention. Addressing Chronic Disease through Community Health Workers: A Policy and Systems-Level Approach. 2nd ed. April 2015. Available at http://www.cdc.gov/dhdsp/docs/chw_brief.pdf.
32. Braun KL, Kagawa-Singer M, Holden AE, Burhansstipanov L, Tran JH, Seals BF, Corbie-Smith, Tsark JU, Harjo L, Foo MA, Ramirez AG. Cancer Patient Navigator tasks across the care continuum. J Health Care Poor Underserved. 2012;23(1):398–413.
33. Patient Navigator Grants. 42 USC §256a. Available at http://www.gpo.gov/fdsys/pkg/USCODE-2010-title42/pdf/USCODE-2010-title42-chap6A-subchapII-partD-subpartv-sec256a.pdf.
34. Harold P. Freeman Patient Navigation Institute. About Us. Available at http://www.hpfreemanpni.org/about-us/.
35. Whitley EM, Drisko J, Everhart RM, Samuels BA. Standardized academic education prepares competent community health workers. Am J Health Stud. 2007;22(2):121–6.
36. Department of Health and Human Services. National Strategy for Quality Improvement in Health Care: 2012 Annual Report to Congress. Available at http://www.ahrq.gov/workingforquality/nqs/nqs2012annlrpt.pdf.
37. Allen JK, et al. Disparities in women's referral to and enrollment in outpatient cardiac rehabilitation. J Gen Intern Med. 2004;19(7):747–53.
38. Scott LB, et al. Examining the effect of a Patient Navigation intervention on outpatient cardiac rehabilitation awareness and enrollment. J Cardiopulm Rehabil Prev. 2013;33(5):281–91.
39. Rosenthal EL, Brownstein JN, Rush CH, et al. Community health workers: part of the solution. Health A. 2010;29(7):1338–42.
40. Anthony S, Gowler R, Hirsch G, Wilkinson G. Community health workers in Massachusetts: improving health care and public health. Boston (MA): Massachusetts Department of Public Health; 2009. Available at http://www.mass.gov/Eeohhs2/docs/dph/com_health/com_health_workers/legislature_report.pdf.
41. National Cancer Institute National Community Cancers Program (NCCCP). Available at http://ncccp.cancer.gov.
42. Department of Health and Human Services. National Institutes of Health. National Cancer Institute. Applied Research: NCCCP. Available at http://appliedresearch.cancer.gov/areas/qoc/ncccp/.
43. Halpern MT, Spain P, Holden DJ, Stewart A, McNamara EJ, Gay G, et al. Improving quality of cancer care at community hospitals: impact of the national cancer institute community cancer centers program pilot. J Oncol Pract. 2013;9(6):e298–304.
44. Ursan ID, Krishnan JA, Pickard AS, Calhoun E, DiDomenico R, Prieto-Centurion V, et al. Engaging patients and caregivers to design transitional care management services at a minority serving institution. J Health Care Poor Underserved. 2016;27(1):352.

45. A Comparative Trial of Improving Care for Underserved Asian Americans Infected With HBV. Project Information. Available at http://www.pcori.org/research-results/2014/comparative-trial-improving-care-underserved-asian-americans-infected-hbv.
46. Moore KJ. An ounce of prevention. Fam Pract Manag. 1998;5(4):12.
47. Moore KJ. Billing medicare for diabetes self-management training. Fam Pract Manag. 1999;6 (4):10.
48. National Conference of State Legislature. Diabetes Health Coverage: State Laws and Programs. 10 Jan 2016. Available at http://www.ncsl.org/research/health/diabetes-health-coverage-state-laws-and-programs.aspx.
49. H.R. 6521—112th Congress: To provide payment for Patient Navigator services under title XIX of the Social Security Act. www.GovTrack.us. 2012. Available at https://www.govtrack.us/congress/bills/112/hr6521.
50. Wells KJ, Battaglia TA, Dudley DJ, et al. Patient Navigation: state of the art, or is it science? Cancer. 2008;113(8):1999–2010.
51. Minnesota Community Health Worker Project. Available at http://www.health.state.mn.us/ommh/projects/chw.html.
52. Minnesota Office of the Revisor of Statues. MS 256B.0625, Subd. 49.
53. Health Homes, Medicaid.gov, Available at: www.medicaid.gov/Medicaid-CHIP-Program-Informaon/By-Topics/Long-Term-Services-and-Supports/Integrang-Care/Health-Homes/Health-Homes.html; see 42 U.S.C. § 1396w-4; 2010.
54. Rabbani R, Wang R, Grasso J. Community health workers and the affordable care act: recommended advanced payment models for employment within healthcare reform programs. Presentation. Available at http://www.swctahec.org/wp-content/uploads/2015/02/CHW_conf_10_sustainable_payment_models.pdf.

Index

Note: Page numbers followed by *f* and *t* indicate figures and tables, respectively

E.A. Calhoun and A. Esparza (eds.), *Patient Navigation*,
DOI 10.1007/978-1-4939-6979-1

MIX
Papier aus verantwortungsvollen Quellen
Paper from responsible sources
FSC® C105338

If you have any concerns about our products,
you can contact us on
ProductSafety@springernature.com

In case Publisher is established outside the EU,
the EU authorized representative is:
Springer Nature Customer Service Center GmbH
Europaplatz 3, 69115 Heidelberg, Germany

Printed by Libri Plureos GmbH
in Hamburg, Germany